The International Behavioural and Social Sciences Library

CHRONIC SCHIZOPHRENIA

TAVISTOCK

The International Behavioural and Social Sciences Library

MENTAL HEALTH
In 8 Volumes

I	Studies on Psychosis *Thomas Freeman*
II	Chronic Schizophrenia *Thomas Freeman, et al.*
III	Mental Illness in the Community *David Goldberg and Peter Huxley*
IV	Mental Illness in Childhood *V L Kahan*
V	Psychological Illness *E J R Primrose*
VI	Mental Health in a Changing World *Edited by Kenneth Soddy and Robert H Ahrenfeldt*
VII	Mental Health and Contemporary Thought *Edited by Kenneth Soddy and Robert H Ahrenfeldt*
VIII	Mental Health in the Service of the Community *Edited by Kenneth Soddy and Robert H Ahrenfeldt*

CHRONIC SCHIZOPHRENIA

THOMAS FREEMAN,
JOHN L CAMERON AND
ANDREW McGHIE

Routledge
Taylor & Francis Group
LONDON AND NEW YORK

First published in 1958 by
Tavistock Publications Limited

Published in 2001 by
Routledge
2 Park Square, Milton Park, Abingdon, Oxfordshire OX14 4RN
711 Third Avenue, New York, NY 10017

First issued in paperback 2014

Routledge is an imprint of the Taylor and Francis Group, an informa business

British Library Cataloguing in Publication Data
A CIP catalogue record for this book
is available from the British Library

Chronic Schizophrenia
ISBN 0-415-26450-2
Mental Health: 8 Volumes
ISBN 0-415-26511-8
The International Behavioural and Social Sciences Library
112 Volumes
ISBN 0-415-25670-4

ISBN 13: 978-1-138-88266-9 (pbk)
ISBN 13: 978-0-415-26450-1 (hbk)

Chronic Schizophrenia

THOMAS FREEMAN
M.D., D.P.M.
Lecturer in Psychotherapy
Department of Psychological Medicine, University of Glasgow
Consultant Psychiatrist, Glasgow Royal Mental Hospital

JOHN L. CAMERON
M.B., CH.B., D.P.M.
Staff Member, Chestnut Lodge Sanitarium, Rockville, U.S.A.
Late Research Assistant, Department of Psychological Medicine
University of Glasgow

ANDREW McGHIE
M.A.
Senior Clinical Psychologist, Glasgow Royal Mental Hospital
Late Research Psychologist
Department of Psychological Medicine, University of Glasgow

PREFACE BY ANNA FREUD

FOREWORD BY T. FERGUSON RODGER

TAVISTOCK PUBLICATIONS

First published in 1958
by Tavistock Publications Limited
2 Park Square, Milton Park, Abingdon, Oxon, OX14 4RN
Second impression 1965

Contents

ACKNOWLEDGMENTS

The authors would like to express their gratitude for the help and encouragement which they have received from Mrs. Dorothy Burlingham, Dr. A. MacNiven, Professor T. Ferguson Rodger, and Professor E. Stengel. Our thanks are also due to Miss M. McDonald who had the arduous task of typing the manuscript.

Preface

It is a special merit of this book that it offers more than the sober title leads us to expect. The authors themselves describe their efforts as a 'clinical, interpretative, and therapeutic study of schizophrenia.' They address themselves primarily to those who—like themselves—work with chronic, hospitalized, severely deteriorated schizophrenic patients, and they make no claim for wider application of their findings. This modesty on their part, on the other hand, should not obscure the fact that readers from many other fields of work can derive profit and stimulation from the careful clinical descriptions and challenging theoretical considerations of this monograph.

In Chapter Two, for example, the theory of mental functioning ostensibly serves the purpose only of providing a theoretical framework—taken from psycho-analysis—against which the authors wish their clinical observations to be viewed. But, beyond accomplishing this task, the chapter provides also valuable instruction for all psychiatrists who are interested in the analytical approach to mental illness, whatever their specific range of case or treatment. It will be welcomed as well by students of psycho-analysis proper as an exceptionally clear and succinct summary of certain basic principles of psycho-analytic thinking.

Chapters Six to Nine are relevant for all workers in the field of analytic psychology. Here, the authors use the severe deteriorations of personality structure, as they occur in the chronic schizophrenic, to discuss in detail those primitive levels of mental life where the distinction between the self and the environment is lacking, with disastrous results for such important functions as perception, thinking, memory, etc. Here students of ego-psychology are presented with vivid clinical pictures of the disturbance of the normal, conscious thought-processes and of their lowering to the level of the 'primary process,' *i.e.,* to that form of mental functioning which normally reveals itself in dream-activity only. Further, the authors show in detail how the 'confusion of identity,' which results from this state of mind, destroys the individual's attachment to his environment and substitutes the most primitive processes of 'merging with the object' for the normal, adult forms of emotional relationships.

In Chapter Ten, finally, readers are introduced to the painstaking methods by which the patients are induced—wherever possible—to re-establish contact with the environment. Child-analysts, and other workers with young children, will note with interest that the therapeutic tools used and recommended by the authors are in many respects identical with the methods used in the upbringing of infants. In the young infant—as in the schizophrenic patient—we find egocentric, autistic behaviour, together with confusion between himself and the environment, both corresponding to a state 'before the boundaries between the self and not-self are adequately formed.' The infant acquires this distinction through his attachment to stable, need-satisfying, reliable figures in the outside world. It is the identification with and introjection of such figures that enables him to build up his ego and sets him on the path to normal functioning.

The authors show convincingly that the formation of such stable relationships is indispensable in the therapy of chronic, institutionalized schizophrenic cases, and they describe in what ways they themselves and, above all, members of the nursing staff were able to serve as figures of this kind.

ANNA FREUD

Foreword

In 1953 The Scottish Hospital Endowments Research Trust, through the Advisory Committee on Medical Research of the Department of Health for Scotland, agreed to finance an investigation into the problems presented by the chronic, hospitalized schizophrenic patient. The research team comprised a psycho-analyst with considerable experience in clinical psychiatry, a clinical psychiatrist whose principal interest lay in clinical research, and a clinical psychologist who was particularly interested in the relation between normal and psychotic processes. The work was carried out at Glasgow Royal Mental Hospital through the good offices of Dr. Angus MacNiven, the Superintendent of the hospital, and consisted of an attempt to study the patients against the background of the hospital environment. A number of methods were employed to achieve this aim.

Although each of the authors brought to the problem his own particular background of experience, the result has been a happy blend in theoretical orientation. This co-operative venture has not only demonstrated how much common ground exists between the disciplines of Psycho-Analysis, Clinical Psychiatry, and Psychology, but also that a conceptual synthesis may be achieved without sacrificing the independence inherent in the different approaches.

One of the most important practical issues raised by this work is the rôle of the mental nurse. This study clearly illustrates the decisive therapeutic influence which the nurse has on the chronic patient. The authors show how this therapeutic potential may be utilized within a framework of the mental hospital.

The success of this investigation was in no small part due

to the co-operation and assistance extended by Dr. MacNiven, and the medical and nursing staff of Glasgow Royal Mental Hospital.

T. FERGUSON RODGER
Professor of Psychological Medicine
University of Glasgow

CHAPTER ONE

Introductory

This monograph is devoted to a clinical, interpretative, and therapeutic study of chronic schizophrenia. It is unnecessary to emphasize the importance of studying this group of mentally ill patients forming as they do a high percentage of the permanent residents of all mental hospitals. The patients who were the object of this study can be roughly divided into two groups. First, those whose personality had deteriorated to a state of 'dementia,' and second, those who, while retaining a considerable degree of personality integration, suffered from fixed delusions of a paranoid type. The clinical features which the two groups presented correspond roughly to some of the nine end states which Kraepelin described in schizophrenia. A brief clinical description of each patient mentioned later in this work is to be found in Chapter Four.

In this monograph we hope to describe both a psychological analysis of chronic schizophrenic symptoms and a psychological method of treatment and rehabilitation. We acknowledge the validity and value of the organic approach to the understanding and treatment of schizophrenia, but we believe that to-day the psychological view, with all its limitations, is in a position to furnish a more integrated and more consistent theory of chronic schizophrenic manifestations, a theory moreover which offers the possibilities of a rational, non-empirical therapy. The theory is not new; it has been available for more than forty years but, apart from Federn's work (1953), few efforts had been made until recently to apply these ideas to the treatment of patients. During the past fifteen years, however, several case reports, *e.g.*,

Sechehaye (1951), Rosenfeld (1954), have appeared which describe therapeutic endeavours.

METHOD OF STUDY

The approach to the schizophrenic patient adopted in the hospital where this work was conducted was based not only upon Kraepelinian nosology but also upon the dynamic theories of Bleuler and Meyer. This was reflected in the routine case notes which were replete with detailed clinical data describing the patient's speech and behaviour. A view of mental illness that regards the symptomatology as a reaction pattern to adverse environmental circumstances or psychological stress demands a longitudinal study of the patient which must embrace the significant experiences of the individual's life. The patient's entry into hospital results in his being exposed to a new set of social forces to which he reacts in his own unique manner. Traditionally this approach is founded upon the relationship between patient and psychiatrist. The impact of environment, both past and present, is discussed within this relationship as part of the treatment situation.

We might now consider the psycho-analytic approach to mental disease which also places great emphasis upon the interaction of the individual and his environment. Here too the approach might be described as both individual and longitudinal. While the Meyerian approach and psycho-analysis take cognizance of the great influence of interpersonal reactions, the individual nature of the treatment precludes consideration of the moment-to-moment experiences of the patient except where these may appear in the doctor-patient relationship (transference).

We have attempted to utilize and apply the insights of psycho-analysis to the study of chronic schizophrenic patients in a group setting. We hoped that by studying the patient in his relationships to other patients, to his nurses and his doctors, it would be possible to observe those conditions attendant upon the emergence, persistence, and disappearance of clinical phenomena. Such observations, we hoped, would also help us to discern the psychological mechanisms accompanying the manifest behaviour. Our aim throughout this work has been to study and treat the schizophrenic patient as a living individual acted upon by interpersonal forces that promote or impede recovery.

We employed three interrelated methods during the two years of study. Our project began with an attempt to influence our chronic patients by means of group psychotherapy. There were two groups, one male, the other female, each containing six patients.[1] The groups met for approximately one hour on four days per week. At the outset it was difficult to know how the patients would react to this novel situation and whether they would interact with one another. As the months went by, in spite of much activity by the patients, we came to the conclusion that there was no evidence of group formation and that they were still behaving as a number of isolated individuals. Nothing appeared at all reminiscent of the phenomena to be found in a group of psychoneurotic patients. A feature of other therapeutic groups is the expression of themes and aims shared by all members. Sustained conversation between the schizophrenic patients never occurred and this precluded the emergence of common aims and ideas, and of differing opinions. It was always possible, of course, that the patients as a group were attempting to push forward some specific problem, but we were never able to grasp it. Indeed, the absence of rational verbal communications soon made us realize that whatever we might infer from the patients' speech and behaviour must remain speculative.

We were confronted at the beginning with a problem—what means were we going to employ in trying to communicate with the patients. Should we forgo confronting a patient with some comment or interpretation of his behaviour because we feared it might be untrue, or should we advance it in the hope that it would at least be a means of contact? In general we inclined to the second course and made interpretations while not giving up

[1]The criteria for selection of the patients are given in Appendix A.

our self-critical attitude. With a few extremely withdrawn patients—some who had not spoken for years—this method was extremely successful for a short time. In retrospect we can say that at the beginning of our work lack of experience and understanding of chronic schizophrenia made us overestimate the value of the spoken word for these patients.

It would give an erroneous impression of the group sessions if we did not emphasize that, in spite of the lack of understandable communications, many of the patients reacted in a most lively and spontaneous fashion. This was true of a number whose condition could only be described as deteriorated in the extreme. This activity was apparent from the early group meetings and was not a reaction to any specific statements on our part. We hope to show later that indeed much of this behaviour was an outcome of the patients being in close proximity with the members of the hospital staff. The patients' reactions provided some of the raw material for a psychological study of chronic schizophrenia and for subsequent treatment recommendations. Later, in Chapter Five, many of the clinical phenomena which were encountered during the group sessions will be presented.

Our purpose in describing such clinical incidents is to underline and confirm certain theoretical formulations which gradually emerged during our contact with the patients. It is worth describing here the method used to gather the clinical material, from which the examples given throughout our later discussions have been selected. During each group session the observer compiled a verbatim note of the verbal and, as far as possible, the non-verbal behaviour, of both patients and therapists. A similar record was compiled during all discussions held with the nursing staff. The separate statements made by patients during the group sessions were finally typed on individual cards in order to facilitate comparative matching of the reactions of different patients and to study changes in a patient's behaviour throughout the running of the groups. All clinical incidents related throughout this monograph are derived from this source. This method of describing isolated clinical examples has been criticized on several counts. Mainly it can be argued that the clinical example selected is influenced by preconceptions deriving from the observer's observational frame of reference.

We believe that much of this criticism ignores the fact that an observer must have some theoretical framework by means of which he can order his clinical observations. With it he is subject to a certain bias; without it he is overwhelmed by a meaningless mass of clinical data. The assumption of a theoretical standpoint must bias the observer to some extent, but the recognition of this factor can lead to a diminution in error. While a complete record of each interview appears desirable, further thought reveals that such records do not solve the difficulty to any appreciable extent. If an independent observer scrutinizes the verbal and behavioural material of the interview as revealed by a record, he too will see it through his own theoretical 'spectacles.' As a result he will agree with the relevance of the significant observation, or he will reject it as meaningless, or advance some alternative explanation of the phenomenon in question.

If we assume that the independent observer believes that there is a meaning in what confronts him, then we are faced with a new problem. This arises from the fact that several psychopathological systems vie with one another in explanation of clinical phenomena. One clinical observation can be interpreted in many different ways. To arrive at a partial solution of this almost insuperable obstacle in present-day clinical psychiatric research, we decided to avoid complex psychopathological inferences when presenting our clinical examples. The decision to do this freed us from the necessity of presenting long accounts of group interviews whose only function would be to decide whether or not a psychopathological explanation of the material was correct. Rapaport (1951) has drawn attention to this whole problem. He points out that although the method of selecting the spontaneous productions of schizophrenics, with the intention of making inferences from them, is fraught with methodological difficulties, it is the method *par excellence* of clinical research. He states (1951) 'Its inherent postulate is the fundamental lawfulness of the biological individual; its inherent danger lies in the difficulty of knowing the realm of applicability of the inferences drawn from the sample chosen.'

The second of the three methods which we utilized to observe chronic schizophrenic patients was originated by Dr. R. D. Laing (see Cameron, Laing, McGhie, 1955). He placed a number of chronic female schizophrenic patients in a pleasant room with two nurses. The patients spent the whole day in this room where they were provided with various occupational materials. The patients were drawn from the crowded female refractory ward where the nursing personnel rarely exceeded five or six. Dr. Laing's intention was to observe the impact, if any, of the new environment, and of the closer contact between nurses and patients. He obtained information about the activities of the group first through a weekly discussion with the nursing staff. This was soon afterwards integrated with the existing meeting conducted for the nurses attending the analytic groups. Second, he spent about an hour daily in the room participating in the work and observing directly. When Dr. Laing left to go to another hospital the management of the treatment centre devolved upon us. Some modifications were made. Our intention was to use the treatment centre as a proving ground for therapeutic measures developed from our observations in the groups. To do this we made our visits as brief as possible in the further hope that the patients would make their requests for favours etc. only to the nurses. The main control was exercised through the weekly meetings, which will be described in Chapter Ten. The nurses soon became extremely interested in the work and they provided a great deal of useful information. The group patients in the centre provided new material which made much of their behaviour in the group sessions more comprehensible. We soon realized that reports of the patients' reactions to the interviews were now available through the medium of the nurses in the treatment centre. A two-way channel of communication was gradually established between the group sessions and the treatment centre. Information from the nurses was available for use in the group sessions and the reactions of the patients were carried to the treatment centre and manifested there. An account of the further development of the treatment centre will be found in Chapter Ten.

The third method of observation consisted in one of us spending several hours per day in the female refractory ward of the hospital. This ward contained approximately seventy patients and at most not more than six nurses. The observer spent a period of from one and a half to four hours daily in the ward where he used to sit in the same seat. He did not interfere in any direct way with the ward management, but never rejected any approach by patients or staff. An important event was the nurses' tea-break to which he was invited. The nurses and he would then discuss events in the ward much as was done at the weekly staff meetings. Full reports of the events in the ward and of the subjects discussed with the nurses were dictated daily.

The work reported in this monograph developed during a two-year project devoted to an enquiry into the possibilities of the psychological treatment and rehabilitation of chronic hospitalized schizophrenic patients. The initial effort consisted of group psychotherapy of two groups of patients, one male and the other female. This was later supplemented by the institution of the treatment centre to be described later.

This monograph is divided into eleven chapters. Chapters Five to Ten contain the kernel of our work, which consists of a psychological analysis of chronic schizophrenic manifestations and a description of a method of treatment and rehabilitation. To enable the presentation of these contributions to achieve the maximum degree of clarity we have prefaced them first with a general account of the psycho-analytic conception of mental functioning, and second with a review of the psychopathology of schizophrenia. We hope that the material contained in Chapters Five to Ten will furnish the justification for our preference for the psycho-analytic frame of reference.

CHAPTER TWO

A Theory of Mental Functioning

The experience of physical medicine has been that the most fruitful studies of abnormal states have occurred when there has been available a relative understanding of normal functioning. Psychiatry and psychology have struggled hard to find the tangible and concrete information that physiologists and pathologists have gleaned in their work with healthy and diseased subjects. Unfortunately the subject matter of psychiatry and psychology has placed wellnigh insuperable obstacles in the path of the fulfilment of this ambition. It has not, as yet, been possible to isolate, measure, and witness the interaction of forces necessary for the performance of a particular mental function. This enormous difficulty has resulted in two divergent tendencies in psychiatric and psychological investigation. While both these trends are complementary, present-day deficiencies in knowledge emphasize the differences rather than the similarities. The first pursues the methods of physiology, biochemistry, and pathology. The second has abandoned this approach, and attempts to comprehend the phenomena presented by abnormal mental states by means of hypotheses that are themselves based upon the behaviour and utterances of the subject under investigation. These hypotheses are essentially psychological.

Freud is an example of those who gave up the physiologico-pathological approach in preference for the psychological view of mental illness. For many years (1894–1900) he tirelessly attempted to utilize his neurophysiological knowledge to unravel the problems of mental disease. He eventually realized that psychological theories were more in line with the clinical findings than abstruse physiological hypotheses that did not even have the backing of observed data. While Freud recognized the immediate value of the psychological approach, he maintained to the end his belief in the physical nature of mental phenomena. He stated (1940) 'The phenomena with which we have had to deal do not belong only to psychology; they have also an organic and biological aspect . . . .' This quotation reveals Freud's insistence that psychological theories should be at all times related to biological function. As a counterpart to this emphasis on the unity of biological and psychological forces he went to great lengths to remove ambiguity by consistently differentiating between biological and psychological concepts. Rapaport reminds his readers that physicists who have become interested in biology have expressed the view that '. . . biological phenomena can be expressed—and already have been, as in genetics—by valid biological laws, despite our ignorance of the underlying and mediating physico-chemical processes. Actually, these views expressed by physicists are quite like the arguments of molar behaviourists, and seem to hold for psychology also.'

One of Freud's greatest contributions has been his description of the two entirely different types of mental activities existing within the mind. Recently Rapaport (1951) has undertaken the task of describing the psycho-analytic concept of the mind. This is, to use his own phrase, a purely psychological model. He believes that the psycho-analytic model is sufficiently flexible to meet the demands which other conceptual schemes were designed to meet. The psychological model has the advantage of being able to integrate psychological observations on their own terms. '. . . the conceptual model implicit to psycho-analysis is sufficiently broad and flexible to embrace on the one hand those realms of psychological phenomena which other models effectively conceptualize, and on the other hand those realms which have remained intractable to them' (Rapaport, 1954).

THE MENTAL APPARATUS

The clinical manifestations of mental illness can best be understood if viewed against the background of the psycho-analytic conception of the mind. The psycho-analytic theory has its origin in Chapter 7 of the *Interpretation of Dreams* (1900). At the outset Freud states: 'I shall entirely disregard the fact that the mental apparatus with which we are here concerned is also known to us in the form of an anatomical preparation, and I shall carefully avoid the temptation to determine psychical locality in any anatomical fashion. I shall remain upon psychological ground, and I propose simply to follow the suggestion that we should picture the instrument which carries out our mental functions as resembling a compound microscope or a photographic apparatus, or something of the kind.' This 'apparatus' which Freud proposed was heavily influenced by his neurophysiological interests and the extent of this influence has been revealed in the letters and drafts he sent to Wilhelm Fliess (1892–1899). In the construction of his hypothetical apparatus he employed his knowledge of the dynamic theory which had then illuminated the study of physiology (*e.g.*, the work of Ludwig, Bernard, etc.). His thinking was in terms of function rather than structure, dynamic rather than static, and was dominated by concepts of functional systems within which conflicting forces met and established ever new equilibria. When discussing the fact that the mental apparatus must be thought of as consisting of a number of systems that may stand in a regular spatial relationship to one another, he goes on to say (1900) 'Strictly speaking there is no need for the hypothesis that the psychical systems are actually arranged in a spatial order. It would be sufficient if a fixed order were established by the fact that in a given psychical process the excitation passes through the systems in a particular temporal sequence.' For Freud it was a matter of 'psychical processes' which dictated the final order of the systems within the apparatus rather than that the processes themselves were determined by a rigid, unchanging structure. All this is very reminiscent of modern conceptions of physiological function—the organ, be it kidney, heart, or lung, adapts to the predominant process occurring within it.

Freud believed that the mind, if reduced to its simplest elements, could be likened to a simple sensori-motor apparatus. Perceptions were registered at the sensory end while neuromuscular activity was initiated at the motor end. Freud utilized this conceptual scheme to explain the visual (hallucinatory) quality of dreams. In his opinion, during sleep the 'excitatory' activity (the neuro-physiological function underlying the psychical process) no longer attempted to reach the motor end of the apparatus but rather moved in a reverse direction finally to reach the perceptual system. In waking life such a regression (*i.e.*, as distinct from the normal progressive direction of psychical processes) to the perceptual system is impossible.

The infant is the subject chosen by Freud to illustrate the earliest stages of the mental apparatus in action. One basic assumption is necessary—that the apparatus has an inherent tendency towards minimizing the degree of internal stimulation. To achieve this end any accumulation of 'excitation' immediately seeks discharge via the motor system. Metabolic processes result in the infant's mental apparatus being suffused with stimuli from somatic sources. The hungry baby can only obtain relief by an actual experience of satisfaction. The perception of the satisfactory experience registered as a 'mnemic image' becomes permanently tied with the memory trace of the need. On the next occasion of hunger there will be a tendency to revive the memory image of the previous gratification and coincidentally an actual re-experience of the perception itself. The movement of 'excitation' arising from the need (hunger) to the final appearance of the perception of the satisfactory experience is a process which occurs during the earliest stages of the development of the mental apparatus. The regressive trend towards the perceptual system of the apparatus is identical with that hypothesized for the dream. Hallucinatory revival, by means of regression, does not by itself abolish the need. This fact must in some way be related to the presence, in the fully developed apparatus, of obstacles that prevent the 'excitation' reaching the perceptual system. This description implied, as Freud went on to show, that two systems operated within the developed mental apparatus. The first attempted to maintain the stability of its *milieu interne* by means of mechanisms already mentioned. The second renounced such measures as the hallucinatory revival of past satisfactions. In its place the second system tried to alter the outside world in such a way as to make real perceptions of potentially satisfying objects possible. The two systems are the forerunners of what were earlier described as the systems preconscious and unconscious. The second system (Preconscious) has at its disposal extensive memory material and the control of motility by means of which it can alter its relationship to the exterior.

Throughout these discussions the concept of energic processes occurring within the mental apparatus is freely used. This is at times referred to as 'quantities of excitation' or as cathectic processes. Such a terminology with its implications of fluctuations in the level of a form of mental energy reflect Freud's difficulty in completely renouncing a physiological background to psychological activity.

Allowing for such considerations, it appears that the first system (named by Freud 'the primary process') is wholly concerned with the immediate discharge of accumulated 'excitatation' irrespective of reality. The second system (named 'the secondary process') prevents this immediate discharge by means of some unknown mechanisms. The charge of energy (cathexis) is rendered 'immobile.' This does not mean that the apparatus has given up the aim of a diminution of tension by means of discharge but merely that this is postponed. During this latent period small expenditures of 'energy' are made in re-awakening the memory systems associated with past satisfactions. This exploratory thought activity, in contrast with the hallucinatory tendency of the primary process, permits the possibility of a final discharge of 'excitation' towards an object in the external world. Freud states (1900), 'The primary process endeavours to bring about a discharge of excitation in order that, with the help of the amount of excitation thus accumulated, it may establish a "perceptual identity" (with the experience of satisfaction). The secondary process, however, has abandoned this intention and taken on another in its place—the establishment of a "thought identity" (with that experience). All thinking is no more than a circuitous path from the memory of a satisfaction (a memory which has been adopted as a purposive idea) to an identical cathexis of the same memory which it is hoped to attain once more through an intermediate stage of motor experiences.'

The study of dreams suggests that the energic processes in the first system (primary process) are wholly different from those in the second system (secondary process). The 'mobile' nature of the cathexes of the primary process has important consequences which are impossible in the secondary process on account of the relatively 'fixed' quality of its cathectic processes. In the primary process 'energy' is freely displaced from one idea to another. The cathexis (energic charge) of numerous ideas may be condensed into a single ideational element. The intense cathexis of the condensation product heightens its sensory qualities and makes it more attractive to internal perception. In secondary process (normal) thinking the importance of an idea to consciousness is not determined by increased sensory vividness. However important a thought may be in normal thinking, this is in no way reflected in an increase in its (sensory) perceptual presentation. The primary process, by nature of its tendency to displacement of 'energy,' facilitates the formation of 'intermediate ideas,' resembling compromises. 'The chief characteristics of these processes is that the whole stress is laid upon making the cathecting energy mobile and capable of discharge; the content and the proper meaning of the psychical elements to which the cathexes are attached are treated as of little consequence' (Freud, 1900). It follows that once ideas whose intensity is heightened because of condensation appear in consciousness they will disrupt whatever train of thought is in process. The presence of intermediate ideas and compromise formations will have the same effect. For this reason processes of this kind are strictly excluded in normal (secondary process) thinking.

DREAM FORMATION

The mental apparatus was conceived on the basis of dream studies. However, it is expedient at this point to reverse the process and utilize the hypothetical apparatus and its mechanisms to illustrate dream formation. The apparatus can be described topographically. It has two principal territories—the system unconscious and the system preconscious. In the former the primary process holds sway, and from it—the borderland between the organic and psychological—emerge the instinctual drives (needs) which attempt to reach the system preconscious. In the latter (Pcs) the secondary process is dominant. In this system ideas of words, which are themselves memory residues, occur while in the system unconscious only the ideas of things (concrete ideas) are present. A barrier exists between the two systems, unconscious and preconscious, and thoughts only become conscious whenever they reach the preconscious. To do this, in Freud's opinion, depends upon the idea of the thing in the unconscious becoming associated with the idea of the word in the preconscious. The preconscious gives both to the instinct drives and other contents of the system unconscious their verbal associations if they are permitted entry into the system. This concept of two systems with their appropriate forces in a relatively unstable equilibrium with one another represents the dynamic aspects of the mental apparatus. A third fact, concerned with the distribution of cathexes (energic charge) is referred to as the economic aspect of the apparatus. A complete description of mental processes therefore demands a topographic, an economic, and a dynamic explanation.

Freud has stated that the principal driving force behind the occurrence of a dream is an unconscious wish. This is in accord with his theoretical view that the unconscious is dominated by the tendency to discharge tension immediately. A second factor contributing towards dream formation is the store of day-time preconscious impressions which continue in the mind during sleep. If by chance one or more of these day-time perceptions has some associative link with the unconscious wish, then the day residue, as it is called, is utilized by the wish as a means of representing itself. As the barrier between the preconscious and unconscious is lowered during sleep, the selected preconscious impressions of the day before are drawn into the system unconscious and there are acted upon by the two main mechanisms of the primary process, *i.e.*, displacement and condensation. Condensation acts in such a way as to compress many trains of thoughts, ideas, and the like into a small number of elements, while displacement results in emphasis being removed from this significant feature to the insignificant features of the dream thoughts. There is a resultant product, the manifest dream, which is quite unlike the latent dream thoughts activated by one or more unconscious wishes. This formation of the manifest dream is completed by a further activity, named 'secondary revision.' While the other mechanisms—condensation and displacement—belong to the primary process, secondary revision is a function of the preconscious. It rounds off the dream and attempts to make it intelligible. The degree of success of the secondary revision is reflected in the rationality of the dream or otherwise. 'There is no doubt, then, that it is our normal thinking that is the psychical agency which approaches the content of dreams with a demand that it must be intelligible' (Freud, 1900).

STRUCTURAL FORMULATIONS

During the years 1900–1919 few radical changes were made in the hypothesis of the mental apparatus. In several papers, 1911 and 1916, many of the issues raised earlier were discussed and elaborated without the occurrence of any significant alterations. However between 1919 and 1923 Freud put forward a new conceptual scheme. This is described at length in *The Ego and The Id*. In this book the human personality is divided into a series of hypothetical mental structures—the ego, id, and super-ego. The id was equated with the system unconscious, the super-ego with the conscience, but with the new knowledge that the conscience had formidable roots extending into the system unconscious. The clinical observation of a 'sense of guilt' without apparent cause, the manifestations of melancholia, and other psychotic reactions supported the super-ego hypothesis. The ego was that part of the personality which was in close contact with the outside world. The ego differed from the id in that it was an organization, whereas the latter was characterized by a lack of integration. The ego was described as the organized part of the id. Freud has said (1923), 'We have formulated the idea that in every individual there is a coherent organization of mental processes, which we call his ego.' The ego had both conscious and unconscious elements. While the awareness of 'self' was a property of the ego, it could not be equated with it. The matrix of the ego was to be found in the multitude of internal and external perceptions which arose from the body, and particularly from its surface. The mental representation of the body ego has been conceived of as the body image.

Clinical psycho-analysis has demonstrated that parts of the ego are unconscious in both a descriptive and a dynamic sense. Descriptive in so far as thought processes in the ego can become conscious without effort; dynamic in that other mental processes are incapable of reaching consciousness because of obstacles standing in their way. These thought processes, which are capable of conscious expression, belong to the system preconscious, which is now considered to be an integral function of the ego. The functions of perception, memory, and control of motility, which were ascribed in the original description of the mental apparatus to the preconscious, were now designated ego functions. Secondary process thinking was, in this new description, a property of the ego. Although elements of the ego extended into the system unconscious the ego maintained, as did the preconscious of the mental apparatus, a barrier against the instinctual drives of the id (system unconscious). While contrary ideas and impulses might exist harmoniously in the id, the ego demanded unity and absence of contradiction. This synthetic power of the ego has been described by Nunberg (1931). Last, but of great importance, is the ego's capacity to test reality.

The ego is the executive agency of the personality. No action is possible unless it enters the system preconscious. Only then might the impulse be translated into consciousness and subsequent action. However, the ego alone does not decide upon the appropriate nature of thought or deed. This is carried out mainly by the super-ego. The ego and id tension remains minimal as long as the former is able to discharge the tensions arising from the instinctual drives in the id. Tension can arise between ego and id, super-ego or reality, hence the concept of conflict between the component mental structures. It is important to note that Freud went to some lengths to ensure that his descriptions of ego, id, and super-ego were regarded only as abstractions. They did not have an anatomical locus nor were they to be looked upon concretely.

Indissolubly connected with the structural concepts of ego and super-ego is the mental mechanism of identification. There are two types of identification—primary and secondary. Primary identification occurs prior to the development of the idea of 'me' as against the 'not-me.' It is suggested that the infant at the breast does not distinguish himself from his mother's body. At this early stage it is difficult to talk of an ego (Fenichel, 1937). Those qualities which are characteristic of the ego (*e.g.*, perception, control of motility) are absent. It is conceivable that there is a kind of pre-ego which is not yet differentiated from the remainder of the psychical apparatus, whose principal function is to abolish excess tension arising from either inner needs or external stimulation. Gradually the infant emerges from the state of primary identification with the surrounding objects. This awareness of a distinction between the self and the not-self is the subjective aspect of the development of the ego boundaries. In maturity these ego boundaries are relatively fixed, while in childhood they remain fluid and unstable. Evidence supplied by several investigators suggests that in the young infant perceptions and motor reactions are 'inseparably intertwined.' Fenichel (1937) quotes Spielrein, Goldstein, and Bernfeld to support this possibility. Goldstein's patients who suffered from brain injuries could compensate for their alexia by following the shape of the letters by movements of their heads. They could read them kinaesthetically, by means of their head movements. Fenichel (*ibid.*) suggests that 'This is a primitive reaction to perception, or rather an assimilation to the percept, a sort of identification, by means of which alone perception can take place. Even though later on what we call "perception" and "identification" are very different, primitive perception is the common matrix of both.'

Secondary identification presupposes the formation of the ego, a realization of the difference between the self and the not-self. In secondary identification permanent changes occur within the ego. These changes take the form of behaving in a similar way to persons who are emotionally important. Childhood is the period when this occurs. Identification with parents and schoolteachers leads to types of attitudes and behaviour similar to that of the objects identified. These identifications occur unconsciously and are dependent upon a satisfactory emotional relationship existing between the child and the adults concerned. In the period when the ego boundaries are not completely settled (*i.e.*, when the me and the not-me are still not completely distinguished), transitory identifications occur which do not last. These secondary identifications may not only have a basis in reality but may have a phantasy root as well. The child may identify itself with imaginary figures which may be pleasurable or frightening. The super-ego is a special example of a structure based on identification. These identifications are normally with the parents but it is important to recognize that important phantasy elements occur in the super-ego development. Often the super-ego is composed of identifications deriving not from the real parents but rather from terrifying phantasy figures. Hence the terror of the super-ego that certain patients show. The super-ego then originates initially from outside impressions, both real and phantasied, and then secondarily becomes 'installed' within the mind.

A new phase in the study of the ego was initiated by Hartmann (1939) in his paper 'Ego Psychology and the Problem of Adaptation.' He pointed out that the clinical material elicited in therapeutic psycho-analysis had underlined the importance of the instinctual drives and the environment as the two main factors in ego development. Conflict between the drives and reality resulted in the appearance of new features within the ego. The process of secondary identification (see above), whereby the structure of the ego is differentiated, is the end result of a conflict between the instinctual drives and the environment. This process has been described by Freud (1923) as follows: 'When it happens that a person has to give up a sexual object, there quite often ensues a modification in his ego which can only be described as a reinstatement of the object within the ego, as it occurs in melancholia; the exact nature of this substitution is as yet unknown to us. . . . At any rate the process, especially in the early phases of development, is a very frequent one, and it points to the conclusion that the character of the ego is a precipitate of abandoned object cathexes and that it contains a record of past object choices.'

Hartmann (1939) found it difficult to believe that every ego function, whose purpose was adaptation to the environment, was a result of conflict. He believed that there must be a conflict-free development of many ego functions amongst which he named—perception, recall, motor development, language, thinking, learning processes, etc. He was careful to point out that this did not mean that these ego functions whose origin was conflict-free might not secondarily be drawn into a conflict situation. Hartmann (*ibid.*) suggested that the term 'conflict-free ego sphere' be applied to those functions 'in so far as they exert their actual effect outside of the realm of psychic conflicts. . . .' Implicit in this hypothesis is the theory that the ego has independent origins. It is not identical in substance with the id even although both may arise from a common 'indifferentiated phase' (*ibid.*). This view had been suggested by Freud (1937) in one of his last papers when he said, 'Our next question will be whether all modifications of the ego (in the sense in which we are using the term) are acquired during the defensive conflict of early childhood. There can be no doubt about the answer. We have no reason to dispute the existence and importance of primary congenital variations in the ego.' During the process of development the ego falls heir to certain inborn equipment. This equipment comprises the perceptual apparatus, the muscular system, etc. Hartmann (1952) states: 'These apparatus as well as those that account for the phenomena of memory, are partly inborn; they cannot be traced, in the individual, to the influence of the instincts and/or reality, and their maturation follows certain laws which are also part of our inheritance.' Those functions which originate in the 'hereditary core' of the ego Hartmann refers to as autonomous factors in ego development. By this he means that these factors enter into the final outcome of the ego as independent variables. This whole hypothesis suggests that any consideration of ego development must take three factors into account. First the impact of reality, second the instinctual drives, and third the influence of the autonomous factors originating in the hereditary material and their maturational laws.

In contrast with the primary autonomy of functions of the ego already mentioned, such as perception, memory, etc., Hartmann has pointed out that there are many other ego characteristics (personality traits, behaviour patterns) which appear to have obtained a relative independence from conflict and regressive tendencies. Here Hartmann means that neither internal nor external stresses result in a deterioration of certain ego traits. This phenomenon gives rise to the question as to what force prevents the disintegration of the ego behaviour into its original form which was derived from the instinctual drive. This tendency towards stability has been named by Hartmann 'secondary autonomy.' In childhood these secondary autonomous factors are most vulnerable. Under stress a newly acquired trait, derived perhaps from some instinctual source by means of a reaction formation (*e.g.*, gentleness instead of cruelty), may give way and the underlying tendency reveal itself. Anna Freud (1952) has pointed to the fact that the stability of the secondary autonomous elements in childhood is dependent upon the object relations. 'Reaction formations that enrich the ego, such as cleanliness, disgust, pity, shame, modesty, or social adaptations such as honesty, fairness, consideration for others, can go by the board in situations when the child's love for the parent changes to hate or hostility or when the bond with the love object is broken. Even as late as adolescence, revolt against the parents is followed by the rejection of identification with them and can lead to reversals of super-ego and ego attitudes, though apparently these attitudes had been fully integrated in the ego structure of the latency child.' The degree of secondary autonomy must vary from individual to individual and it must be of the greatest importance in determining the strength of the ego.

In this brief review of the psycho-analytic theory of mental functioning we would wish to emphasize certain aspects that are particularly relevant to the theoretical formulations which we shall later attempt to develop. In discussing Freud's conception of the mental apparatus we wish to draw attention to his regressive hypothesis which will later be taken up in dealing with the development of hallucinatory activity in schizophrenia. The distinction between the primary and secondary processes together with the concept of secondary revision will also be utilized and developed in our theoretical exposition of the clinical data gathered. Finally, and probably most relevant to our central thesis, is the growth of ego boundaries and the whole function of the ego in the maintenance of contact with reality which, as we will later argue, is so vital in the understanding of schizophrenic thought disorder.

The clinical observations reported in Chapters Five to Nine and the technique of treatment and rehabilitation described in Chapter Ten can be more easily comprehended with the aid of the concepts described above. Schizophrenic thinking, and disturbances of memory and perception, are regarded in this monograph as due to a breakdown in the normal integration that exists between the primary and secondary processes. This does not necessitate a psychological explanation of the breakdown itself. Changes that occur in patients under the impact of the therapeutic regime to be described later in this book are most effectively understood in terms of psycho-analytic ego psychology.

CHAPTER THREE

The Psychopathology of Schizophrenia

During the past two decades views about the psycho-analytic psychopathology of schizophrenia have become increasingly complex and controversial. This has been due to a number of new hypotheses based upon the psycho-analytic study of adult and child patients. We have thought it useful to present this review of the psychopathology of schizophrenia in order to provide a historical background for some of the points that will be taken up later. It begins with the first study of Freud (1896) and concludes with such recent contributions as those of Hartmann (1952) and Katan (1954).

THE PSYCHO-ANALYTIC THEORY OF INSTINCTS

While the last chapter presented a psycho-analytic formulation of mental functioning, any mention of the specific 'material' to be encountered in the mind was omitted. While reference was made to instinct drives and to defence mechanisms, at no point was there an indication as to what the nature of these drives might be or against what the defensive measures of the ego were directed.

According to certain basic assumptions of psycho-analysis the organism is activated by two sorts of instinct drives—the sexual and the aggressive. In his last theory of instincts Freud (1921) named these drives respectively Eros and the destructive instinct.

Their origin is in the id (see Chapter Two), whence they seek satisfaction after finding means of mental representation. Freud conceived that the energy of Eros (libido) had the task of neutralizing the destructive tendencies within the organism. It will soon become apparent that while the earlier psychopathological theories of schizophrenia leant heavily upon the theory of the libido (Eros) this has not been uniformly so with later formulations.

In *Three Contributions to the Theory of Sex* (1905) Freud stated in detail his sexual theory and the correlated hypothesis of libidinal development. As mentioned above, libido was the designation given to the energic processes assumed to underlie the sexual drives. The sexual or libidinal drives are described as having an origin, an aim, and an object. At the beginning of life the libido is wholly concentrated on the rudimentary self. This state of libido distribution is named primary narcissism. This phase of primary narcissism is contemporaneous with that stage, already described in Chapter Two, known as primary identification. There are no boundaries to the self differentiating it from the environment. Concurrently with the development of boundaries there is the tendency for the libido to move outwards and seek objects outside the self. The first object of the infant is his own body. The mother's breast is not appreciated as a separate entity but is felt as an extension of the infant's body. Only gradually does a firm relationship become established with the mother as a completely separate individual. The process whereby this occurs has been described by Hartmann (1952) and Anna Freud (1952). Initially the infant regards the mother only as a means of satisfying basic needs (need-satisfying object) and only later does the mother become an object of constant attention irrespective of immediate libidinal demands (phase of object constancy). The libidinal drives arise from a series of erotogenic zones which in turn dominate the child's libidinal life. In infancy the libido arises from the oral area and the aim of the drives is to incorporate the object—milk, breast, etc. Towards the end of the first year the anal zone assumes greater importance, and the products of the bowel become the object of the libido. The aim of the drives is to retain and control. From the third year onwards the genital region attains primacy and the phallic phase is associated with the series of object relationships known as the œdipus complex. In the period prior to the emergence of the œdipus complex—the pre-œdipal period, the love objects are invested with oral and anal libido and the young child behaves towards these love objects as he felt, or feels, towards the original objects of the drives (*i.e.*, breast and fæces).

During late infancy libido progressively flows from the self to objects. The narcissistic libido gives place to object libido. As the child grows up and successfully renounces the love objects of the early period there is a withdrawal of libido into the ego which has meanwhile been developing. This development, whereby the ego receives a fresh quantity of libido, is termed secondary narcissism to distinguish it from primary narcissism. The withdrawal of libido into the ego from the love objects of childhood is accompanied by the setting up within the ego of these lost love objects. This mechanism is known as secondary identification and has been mentioned in Chapter Two. With the establishment of secondary narcissism a new outflow of libido occurs and there remains after this a reciprocal relationship between the quantity of ego libido and object libido.

In the first weeks the infant obtains libidinal satisfactions from his own body without the aid of an object—this phase of the libido is named auto-erotic. In brief the libido passes through three phases, oral, anal, and phallic, and in each of them the instinct drives have specific aims in relationship to love objects. This orderly sequence of events may be disturbed by the libido becoming 'overattached' to any one phase—*e.g.*, the oral phase may receive a surcharge of libido so that there is a smaller quantity of libido to pass on to the next stage of development. This arrest of libido at any phase is termed fixation. Fixation may be due to two circumstances. First, constitutional predispositions, and second, accidental experiences in early childhood. It is suggested that either over-stimulation or over-frustration of a libidinal zone either oral, anal, or phallic will give rise to a fixation of libido to that area. Associated with the concept of fixation of libido is the concept of regression. Freud has advanced the opinion that if the libido is obstructed in its attainment of satisfaction, there is the tendency for it to fall back to an earlier phase where gratification was obtained. This concept of regression of libido is fundamental to the understanding of symptom formation. Regression involves not only a falling back, *e.g.*, from the phallic phase to the anal phase, but also a regression to the aims and object relationships of that stage. In a similar way the libido may withdraw (regress) from object relationships and return to the ego, augmenting the narcissistic ego libido. In normal circumstances the libido will seek a favourable opportunity to find a new object, but this may not occur if pronounced fixations have occurred during the narcissistic phase of object relationships.

PSYCHOPATHOLOGICAL THEORIES OF SCHIZOPHRENIA

1. *1896–1923*

The earliest psychopathological study of schizophrenia is to be found in the description of a case published by Freud in 1896. He suggested that the repression of childhood sexual (libidinal) experiences determined the content of the symptoms. The delusions themselves were found to be almost unaltered childhood memories while the ideas of reference and auditory hallucinations were regarded as a projection on the environment of the self-reproaches which had followed the infantile sexual activity. Abraham (1907, 1908) made further contributions to this subject. He confirmed (1907) Freud's opinion that if sexual traumata occurred in the childhood of individuals who were later to develop schizophrenia, the content of the symptoms was influenced by these childhood experiences. In the later paper (1908) Abraham suggested that in schizophrenia there is a cessation of object love.

He thought that the patient's libido returned (regressed) to the phase of auto-erotism. In these papers Abraham dissociated his psychopathological explanations from any ætiological considerations. He stated (1907) 'Experiences of a sexual nature, whether they have the true value of a trauma, or produce a less severe impression upon infantile sexuality, are not the causes of illness, but merely determine its symptoms. They are not the cause of delusions and hallucinations; they merely give them their particular content. They are not responsible for the appearance of stereotyped words and postures; they merely determine the form which such manifestations take in an individual case.'

In the next major psychopathological study of the schizophrenic group of disorders, sexual (libidinal) factors were again discovered to be of importance in understanding the delusions of persecution so frequent in these diseases. In the Schreber case (1911) Freud demonstrated that unconscious homosexual tendencies were to be found underneath the delusions of persecution. In this paper he gave a detailed account of the mechanism of delusion formation. It is unnecessary here to discuss the minutiæ of this mechanism beyond saying that an essential feature is the projection of unconscious homosexual trends. Freud proposed in a later paper (1914) that in schizophrenic types of illness there is a withdrawal of libido from object relationships. The libidinal charge (cathexis) is reinvested in the self. This accounts for the megalomanic states so frequently encountered. This narcissistic condition is due to a regression from object love to the narcissistic phase of libidinal development when the individual's love object is his own self. Freud suggested that a fixation at the stage of narcissism must be present in those patients destined to fall ill with paranoia and allied states. In the discussion of the Schreber case (1911) Freud compared and contrasted paranoia with schizophrenia. The latter disease resembled the former in so far as both demonstrated a withdrawal of libido from objects in the external world and its subsequent concentration on the self. In schizophrenia Freud thought the regression of libidinal development extended far beyond the phase of narcissism to the stage of auto-erotism where object relationships are completely absent (see Abraham, 1908). The fixation points for schizophrenia were imagined to be situated further back than in paranoia and to lie somewhere at the beginning of the transition from auto-erotism to object love.

Freud (1911, 1914) advanced the theory that the symptoms of schizophrenia could be regarded as a struggle between the withdrawal and regression of libido from objects and attempts at halting the regression and regaining contact with objects once again. This formulation that envisages two phases in the development of schizophrenia has been utilized by Fenichel (1945) to classify schizophrenic symptoms. Under symptoms of regression in schizophrenia he numbered destruction phantasies, delusions of grandeur, thinking disturbances, etc. Under attempts at restitution he listed delusions, hallucinations, certain catatonic symptoms, etc.

The hypothesis of fixation points, and the concept of libidinal regression to phases appropriate to early infancy, permitted an explanation why certain patients commenced their illness with paranoid symptoms and only later developed all the signs of schizophrenia. Subsequent to the publication of the Schreber case (1911) other reports appeared, *e.g.*, Ferenczi (1914) confirming Freud's theory that delusions of persecution were associated with repressed homosexual tendencies. It is worthy of note that Freud (1911) did not claim ætiological significance for the homosexual libido in delusion formation. He pointed out that unconscious conflicts concerning homosexual tendencies were to be found in the psychoneuroses also. In these patients, who suffered with delusions of persecution, the distinctive feature was the mental mechanism of projection whereby the individual disowned his repressed homosexuality.

Further insight into the psychological mechanisms in schizophrenia was provided by Freud (1915) when he pointed out that in the disease words are subject to the primary process—*i.e.*, to displacement, condensation, compromise formation (see Chapter Two)—in the same way as are the latent dream thoughts. The schizophrenic patient sees a connection between words by virtue of their sound or associative links even though the words denote entirely different things. This suggested to Freud that in schizophrenia the verbal representation of the object was retained intact but not the idea of the object itself. In terms of the libido theory, the verbal idea of the object had retained its libidinal cathexis whereas the idea of the object had lost its libidinal charge. The withdrawal of libido from the idea of the object is but one aspect of the general withdrawal of libido that occurs in the initial phase of the disease (see above). Freud (1915) proposed that it is the attempt at restitution, the tendency to recathect objects with libido that causes the verbal ideas of objects to retain their libidinal investment. In Freud's words (1915), '. . . the cathexis of the verbal idea is not part of the act of repression (the withdrawal phase of the illness) but represents the first of the attempts at recovery or cure which so conspicuously dominate the clinical picture of schizophrenia.'

Between 1919 and 1923 a series of papers was published whose aim was to widen the understanding of schizophrenic delusions. Tausk (1919) identified the 'influencing machine' which occurs in the persecutory delusions of certain schizophrenics as a projection of the body which can be equated with the genitals. Tausk, following Freud's theory of libidinal development, proposed that the delusion of the influencing machine was understandable if viewed as an outcome of libidinal regression to the period of objectless primary narcissism (see above). At this time no boundary line demarcates the self from the non-self and the infant probably regards all sensations as arising from within. Tausk believed that this phase was followed by a projection of all sensations to the exterior coincidental with the outward movement of libido on its way towards objects. One of the first objects the infant finds is his own body. At first this appears not to belong to himself but to the external world. This gives rise to the impression that bodily sensations are coming from outside the self. This experience is repeated in the influencing machine. Tausk points out in his paper that the lack of an 'ego boundary' which differentiates self from not-self in early infancy results in objects being merged with the self and then being discovered over again in the external world. The further development of psychopathological formulations is dominated by this concept of objects temporarily fusing with the self and then reappearing as independent entities, although now bearing some imprint of the previous union.

Nunberg (1921) followed the development of delusions of persecution in a schizophrenic patient. Initially the patient transferred to him (Nunberg) the remnants of his homosexual libido and tried to maintain a relationship with him. As this failed, the patient, abandoning the boundaries of the self, merged himself with Nunberg. From the standpoint of libido theory the patient regressed to the oral phase and incorporated the object. This incorporation (or introjection, which is the psychic correlate of incorporation) revealed itself in the patient's confusion between himself and Nunberg. As a consequence of the loss of boundaries to the self, internal and external perceptions lost their distinctive characteristics. This phase was followed by the appearance of delusions of persecution and ideas of reference. Nunberg became one of the persecutors. Concurrently with this development, the boundaries to the self were re-established and distance was obtained from the object previously 'internalized.' Nunberg observed that the persecutor (himself) was now endowed with the patient's own aggressive and sadistic wishes. Nunberg noted that 'in the phase of projection, objects in the outside world are perceived as such although psychologically they are still parts of the ego.'

In this case Nunberg implicitly associated the mental mechanisms of incorporation (introjection) and projection with a regression of libido to the oral phase. In the initial formulations libidinal regression in schizophrenia was regarded as a withdrawal from objects and a return to the phase of auto-erotism. This hypothesis was mainly concerned with the fate of the libido in terms of object relationships, but in these later studies the regression of the libidinal drives themselves achieved greater prominence. Abraham (1916) pointed out in a case of schizophrenia that the mouth had become the centre of the patient's libidinal interests. A full understanding of the regressive tendencies required a double description—first from the standpoint of the instinct drives and second from the standpoint of object relations. In the former it was assumed that the libido fell back to the oral phase where the aim of the drive was to incorporate (introject) the object. In the latter, occurring simultaneously, there was a return to the phase of primary identification where the absence of boundaries for the self facilitated such processes as incorporation and projection. The concepts of auto-erotism and primary narcissism complemented the description of libidinal regression in terms of object relationships.

An awareness of the leading rôle played by introjection-projection mechanisms in regression to the early days of life (*i.e.*, when the oral zone is the predominant libidinal area) enabled a fuller understanding to be achieved of the mechanisms at work in schizophrenic symptomatology. Nunberg's patient (1921) had introjected the homosexual object and then projected him again, but the projected form had now acquired the patient's own repudiated aggression and sadism. In a similar way the object may be projected but now 'carrying' some physical characteristic of the patient. The machine of the persecutor (see Tausk above) represents a replica of a part of the patient's body. As Fenichel (1945) pointed out, 'Freud's first finding that the persecutor represents the homosexual object certainly remains true; but the fact that the persecutor represents at the same time the subject's own features shows that his object, in the patient's phantasy, had been incorporated and reprojected.' A further development was foreshadowed by the appearance of two papers in 1920 by Van Ophuijsen and Staercke. Both demonstrated that in paranoiac patients the persecutor not only represented a real object but also was perceived unconsciously as the patient's own fæces. While this was in accord with the theory that the persecutor was a reprojected introject, it enabled Abraham (1924) to propose that after the phase of libidinal withdrawal in paranoid types of illness, the patient, as an attempt at recovery, introjected a part of the object. Abraham considered that this oral introjection could occur in other ways than via the oral route and could be thought of as an anal process. Since the discovery of the mechanisms mentioned above, incorporation phantasies in paranoid schizophrenics have been described as occurring via the mouth, skin, and respiratory tract.

2. *1923–1954*

The introduction of the structural approach (see Chapter Two) had no immediate consequences for the psychopathology of schizophrenia. In two papers (1924) Freud transferred the generally accepted psychopathology into the conceptual framework of ego, id, and super-ego. He suggested that in psychosis the ego no longer obeyed the dictates of reality but ignored them in favour of the id. Subsequent developments—*i.e.*, withdrawal from objects and attempts at restitution—followed previous formulations. Some years elapsed before any radical alterations were made in the psychopathology outlined above. All of these later theories utilized the structural approach throughout. In this section only five authorities will be mentioned in any detail because they represent the main trends in the psychopathology of schizophrenia at the present time. Federn (1953), Katan (1954), and Hartmann (1953) advance views which substantially agree with what has been described already, while Klein (1946) and Fairbairn (1944), introduce concepts and hypotheses which differ at many points from the classical psychopathology.

While Federn's explanation of schizophrenia rested upon Freud's theory of the ego (1923), he insisted that the ego is more than a concept. The familiar experience of ego feeling was ample proof of the existence of the ego. Ego feeling allows the individual to differentiate between himself as subject and the outer world, and also between himself as object and all representations of objects. The ego is subject and object in one. Ego feeling was not identical with consciousness, for Federn believed that there were ego states which were not conscious because they had been repressed. In the ego, mental and bodily ego feelings are felt as separated but as nevertheless united in so far as the bodily ego feels the body to be outside, between the mental ego and the environment. The ego was activated by a cathexis (energy charge) derived from libido, from the destructive drives, and from energy arising from the life processes themselves. The ego cathexis invests the periphery of the ego, the ego boundaries. For Federn the concept of the ego boundary is not a static one. He utilizes the term ego boundary to convey the idea that the ego is felt to extend as far as the ego feeling penetrates. 'This feeling sharply distinguishes everything that belongs to the ego in an actual moment of life from all the other mental elements and complexes not actually included in the ego' (Federn, 1953). The ego boundary takes on the function of a sensory organ in order to become aware of everything that goes on outside the ego. What is sensed as thought is a process occurring within the mental and physical ego boundary, what is sensed as real lies outside the ego boundary.

Federn maintains that the ego in schizophrenia is defective because of a weakening of its cathexis. The simultaneous deterioration of the ego boundary results in a failure to differentiate the self from the outside world, in an obliteration of the distinction between the object and its representation by thought (idea of thing and verbal idea—see above), and between preparatory thought processes and subsequent actions. This results in a confused picture of reality resulting in its falsification. This in its turn induces a regression to the ego states of early childhood and infancy together with an inability to utilize abstract thought and an appearance of unconscious mental material. Federn disagreed with Freud's hypothesis that the first phase in schizophrenia was the break with reality and that the falsification of the environment was due to the process of restitution (see above). Clinical observation had convinced Federn that schizophrenia begins not with the loss of external reality but with creation of a false reality as a consequence of the breakdown of the ego boundary. In early cases the therapeutic task was to demonstrate to the patient his falsification of reality and lead him back to an awareness of the environment.

The most controversial and speculative psychopathology of schizophrenia has been advanced by Melanie Klein (1946). Some of this will be seen to bear a close relationship to previous work, while the rest is a complete departure from accepted hypotheses. It is impossible to appreciate her views on schizophrenia without a background of her general theory of mental development. In her opinion, in contrast with classical theory, the infant immediately has a relationship with an object. She does not believe that there is an objectless period—a phase of primary narcissism. The first object for the infant is the mother's breast. The breast becomes the focus of libidinal and aggressive drives (oral-sadistic) —if the breast affords satisfaction, the infant attains the notion of a 'good breast,' which it incorporates. However, if the breast does not afford satisfaction, it becomes the object of violent aggressive tendencies and has the association of 'badness.' The 'bad breast' is similarly incorporated. As a consequence of the aggressive tendencies directed against the external 'bad breast' the infant fears retaliation from it. It equally fears attack from the internalized 'bad breast.' Melanie Klein suggests that from the earliest days the mechanisms of introjection and projection influence the infant's relationship to objects. During these early months the infant has no awareness of a whole object—the mother—but only of part objects which are introjected and projected. An innate knowledge of the penis results in a similar relationship to a 'good' and 'bad' penis which is conceived of as within the mother. This concept of a 'part object'—breast, penis —is derived from the work of Abraham (1924) mentioned above. The introjection and projection of objects, both 'good' and 'bad,' results in the appreciation of reality being influenced by internal psychical activity. The projection of the internal 'bad breast' results in the infant being subject to fears of attack from outside and introjection of the 'bad breast' in its turn results in fears of attack from within. This phase, which is characterized by anxiety resulting from fears of damage, has been named the paranoid position. Klein has made an analogy between the fears of external and internal 'bad objects' and the persecutory fears of the paranoid patient. The paranoid position—occurring about the third month—is followed by the infant gradually becoming aware of the mother as a whole object, and the relationships—both internal and external—that occur at this time have been described as the depressive position. This is however not relevant to the present discussion.

In contrast with Freud's opinion that at the beginning of life no ego exists—*i.e.*, in the sense of the structural hypothesis—Klein (1946) maintains that an ego with effective defence mechanisms is present from the beginning of life. Once again in contrast with Freud's views, Klein believes that the anxiety against which the defence mechanisms are directed is due to a fear of annihilation arising from the activity of the destructive instincts within the organism. According to Klein (1946) the early infantile ego not only lacks cohesion but shows a tendency towards disintegration. The destructive impulses operate from birth and they release defence mechanisms, one of which is a projection of this destructiveness to the exterior where it attaches itself to the mother's breast and thus becomes a source of persecutory anxiety. This projective defence is insufficient to relieve the ego from the threat of dissolution—'under the pressure of this threat the ego tends to fall to pieces. This falling to pieces appears to underlie states of disintegration in schizophrenics' (Klein, 1946). Klein suggests that splitting processes occur within ego and object in order to disperse the concentration of the destructive tendencies. She believes that schizophrenic manifestations may be due to the splitting processes that occur within the early ego as a response to the fear of annihilation. According to Klein's theory, the infant directs anal and urethral drives as well as those of oral-sadism upon the mother's breast and body. In addition to penetrating the mother with poisonous anal and urethral products the infant also introduces into her body those split parts of his ego that are feared and unwanted. This latter mechanism has been named 'projective identification.' Klein (1946) suggests that 'in psychotic disorders this identification of an object with the hated parts of the self contributes to the intensity of the hatred directed against other people.'

Much of Klein's psychopathology of schizophrenia fits in rather closely with earlier theories if allowance is made for differences in terminology. Both views emphasize the role of introjection-projection mechanisms in delusion formation. Such mechanisms are assisted by the absence of a properly defined ego boundary in early infancy. Klein's concept of projective identification is very similar to the concept of primary identification, in so far as the schizophrenic patient confuses himself with his object, discovering repudiated portions of himself in his persecutors. Differences are to be found in the emphasis in earlier theories on the role of repressed homosexuality in persecutory delusions, which Klein replaces by the destructive drives in the genesis of the symptom complex. Again Klein sees in the paranoid-schizoid position a fixation point for later schizophrenic illness, while the classical theory regards the central mechanisms as the initial withdrawal of libido from objects with a regression to the early oral period followed by efforts at restitution.

The other radical revision of psychopathology is due to Fairbairn (1944). In several papers he has introduced a new theory of mental development to replace that of the libido. He maintains that the libidinal drives, erotogenic zones, etc. are secondary to the vicissitudes of object relations. In his opinion (1952), 'Ego development is characterized by a process whereby an original state of infantile dependence, based upon primary identification with the object, is abandoned in favour of a state of adult or mature dependence based upon differentiation of the object from the self.' Schizophrenia, in Fairbairn's opinion, is ætiologically related to the phase of infantile dependence. The emotional conflict in the early oral phase is to suck or not to suck, *i.e.*, to love or not to love. The schizoid individual is afraid of destroying his object through love and for this reason progressively renounces all relations with objects. Fairbairn, like Klein, lays emphasis on the internalization of objects although he differs from her in believing that initially only the 'bad' object is internalized. The schizoid position is the basis for later schizoid and schizophrenic illnesses.

Katan has presented his views on the psychopathology of

schizophrenia in a series of papers (1939–1954). The following brief review of his work is drawn from one of his most recent publications (1954). He has given special attention to two aspects of the schizophrenic illness—first, to the pre-psychotic phase and second to the 'non-psychotic layer' in schizophrenia. The pre-psychotic phase is characterized by a loss of the positive œdipus complex. The boy's attachment to his mother and his ambivalent attitude towards his father is not repressed but has in fact lost its cathexis. The loss of the œdipus complex results in the libidinal drives concentrating upon fixations that are pre-œdipal (*i.e.*, object relations existing prior to the œdipus complex). In the pre-psychotic phase, homosexual tendencies differ from those of the homosexual perversion. The unconscious wish of the pre-psychotic male to be a woman arises not as a defence against the positive œdipus complex but from the constitutional bisexuality of the individual—'. . . in its deepest nature, schizophrenia arises from bisexual conflicts, and this bisexual conflict eventually leads to a state where the heterosexual factor is relinquished' (Katan, 1954). Clinical observation suggests that a certain number of schizophrenic men pass through a narcissistic form of the œdipus complex before the illness breaks out. By a narcissistic form of the œdipus complex Katan means that the boy's love for his mother is partly due to the fact that she embodies his own longed-for femininity. The loss of this narcissistic type of œdipus complex weakens contact with reality and increases the state of narcissism. A struggle ensues to maintain the defence against the unconscious wish for contact with the father (*i.e.*, to behave as a woman towards the father). The father in his turn represents the boy's ideal of masculinity. This narcissistic ideal of the father in the pre-psychotic phase later finds representation in the delusional ideas. In an earlier paper (1950), Katan showed that the God who persecuted Schreber represented part of Schreber himself and God's male organ represented Schreber's genitals. The positive œdipus complex being lost, the individual's only contact with reality is his tie with the homosexual object. This accentuates the unconscious wish for femininity and correspondingly increases the anxiety arising from the fear of castration. The retreat from this danger, and consequently from the homosexual object, results in a break with reality.

Although a patient presents all the characteristics of schizophrenia, this does not mean that the entire personality has become psychotic. Katan concludes that a part of the personality behaves as if the pre-psychotic phase was still in existence. The non-psychotic part of the personality ('the non-psychotic layer') does not remain constant in size but changes all the time. The extent of the non-psychotic layer is dependent upon the activity of the homosexual conflict. If the homosexual urge is not too powerful, the remnants of the ego can function fairly adequately. However, when the homosexual drive increases in intensity, the relative strength of the ego will determine the outcome, *i.e.*, whether or not the subsequent reaction will be in accordance with reality or whether a psychotic symptom will make its appearance. The part of the personality that is affected by the psychotic process regresses to an indifferentiated state where the cathexes of both ego and id are withdrawn. The restitutional phase (see above) allows contact to be restored with reality and the conflict which was resolved by withdrawal is recathected. 'The delusion constitutes the psychotic mastery of a conflict' (Katan, 1954). Katan interprets hallucinations from a dynamic-energic standpoint. He suggests that the energy of the homosexual urge is withdrawn in the psychotic phase, to avoid the danger arising from it, and used to form a hallucination. This releases the tension caused by the homosexual drive and prevents a complete break with reality. This suggests that 'the goal of maintaining contact with reality can be achieved only by abandoning it for a short while through the formation of a psychotic symptom (the hallucination). It is like avoiding a major evil by accepting a minor one' (Katan, 1954).

Hartmann (1953) has employed the concept of neutralization of aggressive and sexual energy in his interpretation of schizophrenia. He describes neutralization as a process whereby instinctual energy is modified and placed at the disposal of the ego. The capacity to neutralize aggression makes it possible for the ego to defend itself against the instinctual drives. In Hartmann's opinion the capacity of the schizophrenic ego for neutralization is damaged. This makes the control of the instinctual drives more difficult. The liberated instinctual energy may be directed against the environment or projected or turned against the self. Many details of schizophrenic symptomatology can be explained with the use of this hypothesis (see Hartmann, 1953).

This review of psycho-analytic formulations regarding the psychopathology of schizophrenia shows that during the past twenty years there has been a tendency for new hypotheses to seek recognition. The relationship of these new theories to the original views proposed by Freud and others varies from a relatively close adherence to a fairly wide divergence. However close or distant such theories stand in relation to the older beliefs, they are characterized by one distinctive feature—the almost universal attempt to derive ætiologically significant hypotheses in purely psychological terms. For example, Bak (1954), who follows rather closely Hartmann's views on the psychopathology of schizophrenia (see above), relates the changes the patient experiences in the self basically to a failure on the part of the ego to neutralize aggressive energy. He states (1954), 'The sudden inability of the ego to neutralize aggression (which inherently means the loss of the object in varying degree) turns the entire aggressive drive loose, and this develops increasing impetus and destroys the self that has become its object.' Bak points to the similarity between his conclusions and those of Klein (1946) who, as has been mentioned above, considers the essential disturbance in schizophrenia as due to the disintegration of the ego—this disintegration (splitting) being in part a defensive reaction of the infantile ego against the destructive drives.

More than any other group Klein and her followers have consistently interpreted every aspect of schizophrenic phenomenology as an expression of underlying psychopathological conflict, without any reference to a disturbance in function of the mental apparatus. For example, Rosenfeld (1950) suggests that confusional states occurring in chronic schizophrenia are due to a predominance of aggressive impulses which results in aggressive and libidinal drives and 'good' and 'bad' objects becoming mixed up. Following the general theory of schizophrenia laid down by Klein (1946), Rosenfeld suggests that the anxiety that often accompanies such confusional periods is due to the danger that the destructive drives may destroy the libidinal impulses, with the consequence of impending annihilation of the self. Again, Bion (1954), in an interpretation of schizophrenic speech, advances the opinion that the schizophrenic patient utilizes language first as a means of projective identification, and second for the purpose of splitting the object. In the former instance the patient uses words as things or as split-off (repudiated) parts of himself which he forcibly pushes into the analyst. In the latter situation splitting of the object is called for when the analyst represents an internal persecutor—this enables the patient to maintain an idealized picture of the analyst to offset his fear of him as a persecutor. The patient's utterances and behaviour are interpreted to him on the basis of these theories.

The earlier theories of schizophrenic psychopathology and those of Hartmann (1952) and Katan (1954) are drawn against the background of the mental apparatus as described in Chapter Two. Thought disturbance, disorders of perception, memory, and reality-testing are regarded as being due to a disorder of function within the apparatus. Freud (1900) believed that the presence of two separately functioning systems within the apparatus—the primary and the secondary process—was a potential source of abnormality. Freud thought that '. . . those, (illnesses) at least, which are rightly named functional do not presuppose the disintegration of the apparatus or the production of fresh splits in its interior. They are to be explained on a dynamic basis—by the strengthening and weakening of the various components in the interplay of forces. . . .' Psychopathological formulations were not initially intended to provide a causal explanation for symptom formation in schizophrenia. The task set for psychopathology was to provide answers to questions quite separate from queries about the basic processes underlying schizophrenic symptomatology. Psychopathology began by trying to explain why a particular symptom occurred in a particular individual, and what determined the content. This led initially to the recognition of the connection between infantile sexual experiences and the content of later psychotic symptoms (Abraham, 1908). This was extended to the appreciation of unconscious homosexual conflicts in cases of paranoia and schizophrenia in general.

During the past twenty years psychopathological theory has gradually ousted the mental apparatus, conceived as an energy system, as a basic concept for the comprehension of schizophrenic symptoms. This trend has reached its climax in the work of Melanie Klein (1946) and Fairbairn (1952). Both lay great stress upon concepts of mental structure (*i.e.*, ego, id, super-ego, internal objects, etc.). This emphasis is reflected in the type of explanation of psychotic symptoms presented by Klein and her followers. The tendency throughout this work is to replace the functional (dynamic-economic) aspects of mental life implicit in the original formulation of the mental apparatus by a concretized system of object relationships. The difference in approach is best illustrated by contrasting the psychological mechanisms conceived of by Klein (1946) to account for infantile hallucinatory gratification with that proposed by Freud (1900) (see Chapter Two). Freud thought that hunger in the very young infant was accompanied by an increase of 'excitation' within the mental apparatus. Previous experience of satisfaction at the breast had resulted in the perception of the need becoming permanently tied to the memory trace of the need. The reappearance of hunger tends to evoke the memory image of the previous gratification and a simultaneous experience of the perception itself. Such an explanation of hallucinatory gratification, which emphasizes the close link between memory trace and perception, has received support from Penfield's work (1952) on the stimulation of the temporal lobes and from the study of the 'imprinting' process in animals by such ethologists as Tinbergen and Lorenz.

Klein (1946) does not believe that such a simple explanation accounts for infantile hallucinatory experience. She assumes that the young infant's mind is capable of what would seem to be complex ideational activity. She believes that by splitting off the frustrating and persecutory aspects of the 'bad' breast (see above), the infant maintains the hallucination of a gratifying experience. The 'bad' breast is not only kept apart from the 'good' breast but is completely denied. Klein states (1946): 'In hallucinatory gratification, therefore, two interrelated processes take place: the omnipotent conjuring up of the bad persecutory object and the painful situation. These processes are based on splitting both the object and the ego.' Schizophrenic symptomatology is thus seen as a consequence of a fixation at a stage of object relations where the infantile ego cannot master the intense anxieties arising from the activity of the destructive instincts.

In our view a general theory of schizophrenia based only on psychopathological content is insufficient to account for similar disturbances in organic and toxic psychoses and in normal subjects exposed to abnormal environmental situations. A general theory must also take into account the functioning of the mental apparatus.

CHAPTER FOUR

The Patients

Before entering into the detailed discussion of the clinical phenomenology in the following chapters we wish to present a brief account of the patients to whom we refer by name. All the patients studied were from the chronic refractory wards of the hospital. An idea of their 'chronicity' can be obtained by considering the duration of their illness and the treatment that had been used.

Among the female patients the average duration of illness was eight years, with a minimum of four-and-a-half years and a maximum of twelve years. Among the male patients the average was nine years, with a minimum of six years and a maximum of nineteen years. The average amount of physical treatment that had been used for both male and female patients was three injections of Cardiazol, seven electro-shocks, and forty insulin-induced comas per patient. At the beginning of the investigation the quantity of sedative being used was considerable and was rather more than one sedative dose per patient per day.

The following short descriptions are based upon the hospital records and upon a brief psychiatric interview before the work began. It will become obvious to the reader that these accounts are very similar to one another. It is our contention that loss of individuality is a feature of the chronic patient in the refractory ward.

THE FEMALE PATIENTS

Emily Smith (*age 26*): Single. Duration of illness: Four-and-a-half years. Previous treatment: Three courses of electro-shock therapy and a complete series of insulin comas. Prior to admission she was a clerkess, and had been a local beauty queen. She was untidy and her clothing was usually torn. There were sores on her face from picking at her skin. In general she gave the impression of being perplexed and puzzled. Often in the ward she would jump up, shout angrily, and shake her fists. Although not regarded as highly dangerous, she occasionally did attack the staff and other patients.

Myra Green (age 29): Single. Duration of illness: Eleven-and-a-half years. Previous treatment: Four courses of electro-shock therapy and a full course of insulin comas. She had been a shorthand-typist. In the ward she was very quiet and did not speak even when addressed. Characteristically she sat on a chair with her knees drawn up, grimacing with one eye closed. She was pale, withdrawn, and untidy, with smeared food and fæces on her clothing. At times she masturbated publicly and used to wash her hair in the W.C. when she had the opportunity.

Jessie Brown (age 35): Single. Duration of illness: Twelve years. Previous treatment: A course of electro-shock therapy. She was a University Honours Graduate in Arts. She was very disordered in her dress and her clothing was usually badly torn. She was continuously in motion, with rapid and jerky movements. She shouted and talked in a manner incomprehensible to the occasional observer.

Cathy White (age 26): Single. Duration of illness: Six years. Previous treatment: Two courses of electro-shock therapy and one of insulin coma. She had previously worked in a food factory. She had been mute for years and, usually, sat motionless, bolt upright with her hands folded in her lap.

Barbara Thomson (age 26): Single. Duration of illness: Four-and-a-half years. Previous treatment: One complete and one incomplete course of insulin coma. She had been a clerkess in the civil service. She was restless in the ward and carried her possessions packed in a bag. If the door was left open she would try to leave the hospital. Occasionally she was successful, and had the reputation of being a 'chronic escaper.' Although her clothing was untidy she used to maintain a brilliant smile and sustain prolonged though superficial discussions which always led up to the subject of her release from hospital.

Betty Jones (age 29): Single. Duration of illness: Eleven years. Previous treatment: Two very prolonged courses of electro-shock therapy. Prior to admission she had been a probationer nurse. She was usually mute and motionless but would occasionally become very angry and shout loudly. Her manner was timid but unfriendly. When approached she would turn away so that her eyes did not rest upon the person who spoke to her.

Mary Bruce (age 43): Single. Duration of illness: Four years. Previous treatment: One course of electro-shock therapy. Often she was aggressive and would attack patients or staff who approached too close to her. She was very noisy and would shout in loud aggressive tones at her 'persecutors.' Her dress was disordered and her clothing usually torn.

Annie Alexander (age 54): Married. Duration of illness: Four years. Previous treatment: One course of electro-shock therapy. She was very suspicious of the staff, and never answered questions. She was noisy, restless, and occasionally threatening. Her clothing was usually torn and disordered.

Jean Tyler (age 46): Divorced while in hospital. Duration of illness: Twelve years. Previous treatment: Three courses of electro-shock therapy. She was an untidy, demented person and her speech was incomprehensible. With the nurses she was suspicious and would not do what they asked her. At times she was very noisy and aggressive.

CHRONIC SCHIZOPHRENIA

Betty Cathcart (*age 32*): Single. Duration of illness: Eight years. Previous treatment: Two courses of electro-shock therapy before a leucotomy operation was performed in 1949. A further course of electro-shock therapy in 1951. She was admitted to hospital from the Women's Auxiliary Air Force. On the whole she was quiet and apathetic though occasionally she would begin to scream for perhaps five minutes. At times she would attack other patients violently. Her clothing demonstrated her complete lack of interest in herself.

Rachel Faith (*age 46*): Widow. Duration of illness: Four years. Previous treatment: Two courses of electro-shock therapy. She had a marked acne rosacea of the face at which she used to pick until it became septic. Her speech was incomprehensible. At times she was violent, attacking particularly the senior nurses. She had a penchant for window-breaking.

Peggy Rait (*age 35*): Divorced while in hospital. Duration of illness: Nine years. Previous treatment: Two courses of electro-shock therapy. She was regarded by the nursing staff as one of their most dangerous charges. She was prone to attack any one and every one. Her speech was incomprehensible, and her appearance dishevelled and disordered.

THE MALE PATIENTS

David Black (*age 36*): Married. Duration of illness: Six years. Previous treatment: One course of electro-shock therapy and one course of insulin coma therapy. He was very disordered in clothing and in manner. His speech was a jumble, and usually incomprehensible. He presented the picture of a restless, grossly demented chronic patient.

James Brown (*age 30*): Single. Duration of illness: Seven years. Previous treatment: One course of electro-shock therapy. He had been employed as a clerk before his breakdown. His clothing was usually untidy as he repeatedly tied and untied his boots and tie, and buttoned and unbuttoned his jacket and waistcoat. He was timorous, and made no spontaneous comments, his speech being restricted to 'Yes,' 'No,' and 'I couldn't say.'

Andrew Gray (*age 30*): Divorced. Duration of illness: Nine years. Previous treatment: Two courses of electro-shock and two courses of insulin coma therapy. In the hospital he spent most of his time working in the kitchen. He made apparently good contact with people about him and his dress and manner were normal. Occasionally he would twist his head sharply to the right and back to the front again, at the same time making a spitting noise with his mouth. He swore obscenely, but would flatly deny that he was responsible, claiming that a machine made him do this.

George Johnson (*age 39*): Single. Duration of illness: Nineteen years. Previous treatment: A course of Cardiazol and a course of insulin coma treatment. He had been of independent means. His clothing was untidy and he was suspicious and unapproachable. His speech was fluent, but was difficult to follow. At times when annoyed he would strike out with such force and accuracy that the victim was usually rendered unconscious.

Dennis Wylie (*age 36*): Single. Duration of illness: Seven years. Previous treatment: One course of insulin shock therapy. He had been a chauffeur-gardener. His clothing showed evidence of care. Normally he was impassive and detached and would sit for hours ignoring what went on around him. When addressed he would reply in a staccato and monotonous voice, usually requesting married quarters for himself and one of the doctors, a lady whom he believed to be his wife.

George Wilson (*age 30*): Single. Duration of illness: Six years. Previous treatment: One course of Cardiazol, two of electro-shock therapy, and one of insulin coma therapy. Prior to his breakdown he had been a commercial traveller. He was detached and uncommunicative, and he only spoke to ask to go to the toilet or for a cigarette. His clothing was untidy. He had an unusual mannerism, twitching his scalp and making his ears move.

CHAPTER FIVE

The Basic Disturbance in Schizophrenia

In Chapter Two we discussed the psycho-analytic conception of the mind or mental apparatus and described the state of primary identification, which appears to be present in early infancy before the ego boundaries are adequately formed. At this stage of development there is no awareness of a distinction between the self and the not-self. This distinction develops gradually as the ego boundaries begin to form, allowing secondary identification to take place. It is a disturbance of the development and maintenance of adequate ego boundaries which, on the basis of clinical observation, we have come to regard as the central feature of the schizophrenic disease process. As this view will be developed and its ramifications considered throughout the remainder of our discussion, it is desirable to define our basic terms in connection with it in as clear a manner as possible. We can do no better than to quote the description given by Federn (1953), who has probably done more than any other person to elucidate and develop the role of ego functioning in the basic picture of the mind laid down by Freud. Speaking first of 'ego feeling,' the subjective aspect of the term 'ego boundary,' Federn says 'Ego feeling is the sensation, constantly present, of one's own person—the ego's own perception of itself . . . This self experience is a permanent, though never equal, entity which is not an abstraction but a reality. It is an entity which stands in relation to the continuity of the person in respect to time, space, and causality. It can be recognized objectively and is constantly felt and perceived subjectively. We possess, in other words, an enduring feeling and knowledge that our ego is continuous and persistent . . . because we feel that the processes within us . . . have a persistent origin within us and that our body and psyche belong permanently to our ego.' It is obvious from his description that Federn regards this 'ego feeling' as a dynamic and living entity, far removed from a theoretical abstraction. With this we would heartily concur, and we hope that the clinical material given later in this monograph will demonstrate to the reader the vital reality and significance of the concept. Federn defines the term 'ego boundary' as follows: 'The term ego boundary shall not designate more than the existence of a perception of the extension of an ego feeling. These boundaries . . . are always changing. But a person senses where his ego ends, especially when the boundary has just changed.' It may be suggested here that these terms enhance what is implicit in such concepts as Rapaport's 'reflective thinking.'

The development of 'ego feeling' and the gradual formation of ego boundaries can be observed in the young infant. Piaget and other investigators of the behaviour of children have illustrated the 'egocentric' behaviour that occurs before the boundary between the self and not-self is adequately formed. Piaget (1928) has vividly described the reality world of the young child who, for example, reasons that the sun does not go away 'because sometimes we don't go away.' Bender and his co-workers, studying sensory phenomena by neurological techniques, report disturbances which they associate with alteration in the body image occurring in normal children of 4 years. Kanner (1949), Rank (1949), and others have stressed the lack of adequate ego discrimination in the group referred to as 'autistic children' or, by others, as 'childhood schizophrenics.'

However, even after the formation and development of ego boundaries, the individual may be exposed to situations in which the boundary between himself and his environment is disrupted. Federn (1953), Silberer (1912), Rapaport (1951), and others have drawn notice to correspondence between elements in the hypnagogic state and the ideational experience of schizophrenics. Federn indeed rather dryly offers the former state as an illustration, available to all, of the elasticity of the ego boundary. 'The hypnagogic change at the brink of sleep consists in the fading away of the ego. This phenomenon gives to every person the opportunity to convince himself of the existence of his ego cathexis and of his ego boundaries, provided he is willing to sacrifice the pleasure of falling asleep normally.' Other investigators have mentioned similar experiences in such states as awakening from anaesthesia, insulin coma, electro-convulsive therapy, reduced states of consciousness due to lack of oxygen in higher altitudes, and many toxic states. Most vivid illustrations of this lapping over of the person into the surrounding environment are provided by the number of recent studies on chemical intoxication produced by such drugs as mescalin, hashish, and lysergic acid. One subject under mescalin, upon hearing mouth-organ music outside declared, 'I am music—I am climbing in music.' Another reported, 'I feel my body floating over without limit into the surroundings.' In such states it would seem that the normal distance between the ego and the external world is almost eliminated (Werner, 1940).

Again, investigators in the organic field have pointed to the weakened sense of personal identity as the basis of the perceptual anomalies seen in cases of organic brain damage. Indeed, Goldstein's (1939) analysis of concrete and abstract thinking is based entirely on this loss of the capacity to 'experience a distinction between oneself and the world' in cases of cortical damage. *It is this factor of 'ego feeling,' or the ability to differentiate the self from the environment, that we regard as being damaged in chronic schizophrenia, thus leading to the patient experiencing internal and external sensations as a continuum. We believe that, once this basic disturbance is appreciated, all other schizophrenic manifestations can be viewed as necessary elaborations of it.*

CHAPTER SIX

Confusion of Identity

The most direct result of the breakdown of ego boundaries is the schizophrenic patient's confusion regarding his own identity. All the patients, at one time or another, gave evidence that they were unsure of their personal identity. They were frequently puzzled and bewildered. One patient said, 'Do I have a face? It's my face. I have a face. Is this my face? There is only one face, one nurse, one hospital.' Another patient, looking similarly bewildered, said hesitatingly, 'Am I a nurse? I'm not a nurse. Am I a doctor?'

Not uncommonly patients referred to themselves in the third person, *e.g.*, a patient said, 'I knew a wreck called Emily.' Individuals who were usually taciturn and refused to answer when addressed directly would sometimes talk in an animated way about themselves in the third person.

While these examples illustrate the patient's failure in self-recognition, the following instances depict their difficulty in differentiating themselves from others. The confusion of patients between themselves and others in their immediate environment was as frequently demonstrated by actions as by speech. One patient, Jim Brown, had been receiving cigarettes whenever he asked for them. One day the therapist had only a few with him, which were quickly exhausted. The patient kept asking for another cigarette although he was informed on each occasion that there were none left. When it was finally suggested that the patient should search the therapist's pockets, Jim promptly went through his own pockets.

When a patient's clothing was dirty, torn, or considered unsuitable by the nurses, they would sometimes dress the patients in another's clothing. This practice, not uncommon in mental hospitals, added greatly to the patients' confusion about themselves. One female patient, Emily, came in one day looking unusually perplexed. She said, 'So I'm Margaret Provost after all.' She was fingering her coat near the hem and one of the therapists, realizing that the coat was not her usual one, looked at the label and found the name 'Margaret Provost.' This kind of reaction was, in the authors' experience, a frequent accompaniment of such clothing changes. Emily Smith had often made references to her dislike of working for her stepmother, *e.g.*, 'I'm not going to work for that old bitch.' These references were often obscure and accompanied by swearing. One day Jessie Brown came in shouting and swearing in a manner unusual in her. She said, 'I'm bloody well not going to work for that old bitch.' The significance of her behaviour was not appreciated at first but Emily kept watching her and finally pointed at Jessie, saying 'She has my coat. She is my sister. My sister has taken my coat.' Jessie replied, 'I'm turning into my sister.' Jessie was in fact wearing Emily's coat. The disturbance which these well-meant changes of clothing produced is best summarized in the words of a patient. She asked, in a puzzled way, 'If I took another frock off somebody who is not me, would I be her?' Again, one is reminded of the similar phenomenon demonstrated by young children where a change of dress can transform the personality completely. Piaget (1951) writes of a boy of 2½ years finding his father dressed in an unfamiliar black suit. Looking at him open-mouthed the child asked, 'What are you now, Papa? Are you Grandpa?'

In general one gets the impression that the patients constantly confuse themselves with anybody, regardless of that person's importance. On one occasion, a maid, who was quite unfamiliar to the patients, came in with a coal-scuttle. A patient said, 'I am the person who brings in coal.' On another occasion a male patient sat beside another who had an explosive oral tic. When the other's tic occurred, he said, 'I'm spluttering.' Psychiatrists have commented on this particular type of confusion but have interpreted it differently. Storch's report (1923) on the verbalizations of his schizophrenic patient provided an extremely clear correspondence with our observations. The patient described his experiences as follows, 'What I was and what you were I often could not tell . . . You and I . . . it's all the same, isn't it?' Another of his patients gave an even more vivid description of the lack of distance between herself and the external world. 'Gradually I am no longer able to distinguish how much of myself is in me and how much is already in others. I am a conglomeration, a monstrosity, modelled anew each day.' The same fear of fusion with others was expressed by one of our chronic patients who declared, 'I have lived with these other people (patients) for so long and we have eaten and drunk together. Now they are all part of me and I am part of them. I'm frightened—I only want to be myself.'

It is essential to pay great attention to this constant tendency on the part of patients to identify themselves with persons in their environment. Much of what is said appears as gibberish unless it is remembered that such transient identifications constantly occur and, indeed, the failure to appreciate this fact may lead to misleading psychopathological conclusions. For example, the female patients often queried their sex in the presence of a male therapist. In an earlier example one patient asked if she was a doctor. She continued: 'Trousers. Each man and woman has trousers on. I have trousers on.' Another patient would frequently stand in front of the fire holding a poker in front of her genitals. When asked about this she said she was 'a man standing up.' This behaviour could be interpreted, and some writers have interpreted it, as evidence of the patient's wish for maleness, instead of recognizing it as another instance of the basic schizophrenic disturbance, namely the breakdown of the ego boundary.

Echopraxia falls into the same category. This phenomenon occurred fairly frequently and was usually transient in nature. For example, one therapist had a habit of slapping his pockets as he looked for cigarettes and matches. When he did this one of the female patients used to slap her own sides as though she were wearing a man's jacket. One of the male patients used to sit imitating every gesture by a particular therapist—his posture as he sat, his movements, and the way he held his head were all a replica of the therapist.

Primary identifications are usually of transient duration as the examples already given demonstrate, but when they occur with people of emotional importance they tend to be of greater duration. By emotional importance no more is implied than availability. When people are constantly in the environment of such patients they thereby become important. If the person makes some attempt to meet the needs of the patient then he becomes sought after and the identification is less transient. Accordingly, identifications with staff as compared with other patients tend to last longer. David Black, one day, was heard muttering remarks addressed to other members of the group. 'It's a mental test. I'll give you a mental test, Mr. Johnson. Speak up now, Mr. Wylie. I'll test you. What's your complaint, Mr. Brown? Yes, I'm a nerve specialist. I'll test you.' He would say he was a doctor, usually a brain specialist, but at other times a heart specialist or a stomach specialist. 'What's your complaint? Speak up now. You are supposed to talk here. It's your heart? Let me see your pulse.' With this he would take hold of the wrist of the person whom he was addressing and count, tap him on the chest as though percussing, and put his ear to the front of his chest. 'Ah, yes, Mr. Brown. It's your nerves. Cross your knees.' This behaviour was sustained for many sessions.

Of marked interest are the identifications that occurred with the nurse. One day the nurse cleaned the nails of some of the patients. The following day Betty Jones adopted a masterful and controlling attitude to the others. When one patient shouted angrily, Betty said, 'You control your temper or I'll manicure you.' Some of the identifications with the nurse led to groping attempts on the part of patients to behave in a manner which led to alterations in themselves or their environment. These alterations were often of constructive type, particularly when the identification was of less transient nature. One of the female patients (Emily), who frequently confused herself with the male therapists, would on these occasions begin to remove hair grips from her hair or take off her stockings, muttering angrily about women's clothing. This type of activity ceased at times when her speech and behaviour indicated her identification with the nurse. This particular nurse had curled hair parted in the centre. Emily, whose hair, if not hanging in disorder, was parted at the side, stared at it, saying, 'You have a centre parting. I have a centre parting. Your hair is curly.' She began to pull her hair over her face with her fingers—quite a usual activity on her part—but instead of leaving it hanging or pushing it back carelessly, she began to part it down the centre. This activity continued for several sessions until one day when the therapists came in she said, 'I have a centre parting.' Her hair was neatly done with a centre parting. She seemed very proud of it and frequently drew the attention of people present to it. During this period many of her statements and actions indicated that she believed she was the nurse. She was much less perplexed and confused and her speech was clearer. Later she became puzzled, 'My hair is curly. Is my hair curly? I am a nurse. Am I a nurse?' When asked if she would like a permanent wave the patient said that she would. The day after her visit to the hairdresser, Emily was very angry. She swore bitterly about the woman who had put her under the machine, shouting finally, 'I'm not a nurse, just a bloody patient.' She pulled angrily at her hair. It was noticed that her permanent wave had not made her hair curly, as she had hoped.

The emotional factors which caused prolongation of these identifications were not always directly concerned with the individual with whom the identification had occurred. One patient, Jessie Brown, had become attached to one of us who was at that time visiting her ward containing seventy chronic patients. During the group session one morning this patient did not respond when the therapist spoke to her by name. Finally she turned to him in an irritated way and snapped, 'I'm Alford. My name is Alford.' The therapist recalled that in the ward that morning he had spent some time speaking to a maniacal girl called Margaret Alford who had been sitting next to Jessie. The patient continued to call herself Alford for several days after this event.

BODY IMAGE

The authors constantly encountered phenomena, of which a few examples are given above, indicating that the perception of the body was seriously disturbed in their patients. One of the authors having heard of Beata Rank's work (1948) with autistic children decided to use physical contact in an attempt to establish communication with two female catatonic patients who had not spoken appreciably for many years. The technique was simple. The therapist stroked the patient's cheek, reiterating, 'This is Cathy's cheek. You are Cathy. This is your cheek. My hand is stroking your cheek.'

The first patient approached, Cathy White, did not respond at the beginning except to flinch slightly. When the therapist stopped, Cathy began to move spontaneously—a most unusual activity. She touched her cheek and studied her hands in a bewildered, puzzled way. The therapist repeated the process and this time the patient became restless. She frowned, caught at his hands and pushed them away. Finally she began to speak. 'You had better go and sit over there,' and she pointed to a chair on the other side. For the next few days as a result of continuing the stroking she became more animated in action and speech. She finally struck at the therapist, afterwards saying, 'I'm afraid when you are close because I cannot see.' The therapist asked, 'See what?' The patient replied, 'You and me.' It was observed during this week that the patient continued to study her hands and body, touching herself all over. The nurses reported that her behaviour was changing. She was in general more active and interested in herself and stood at times in front of the mirror. On one occasion she began to smile and said, 'I think that I'm beginning to see now. I can see you and me.'

The response of the second patient, Betty Jones, to this physical contact was similar but lacked the physical aggressiveness of Cathy. She also touched her cheek and examined, first her hands and later her whole person. Her comments were to the effect that 'I'm keeping an eye on you.'

One might regard these responses to physical contact as a result of the fear of sexual assault. However, the authors are of the opinion that the reaction to the therapist's actions and the improvement that ensued can better be understood on the basis of changes in the patient's ego feeling. The loss of ego feeling also applies to the patient's perception of his body, and in severe psychotics this is disturbed, a symptom to which Federn, among others, has drawn attention. Federn (1953), after describing the withdrawal of the mental ego cathexes in schizophrenia, goes on to discuss the extension of this to one's self-perception of the body. 'There exists still another form of loss of ego boundary cathexes . . . When an inner organ loses its ego cathexes the self-perception of one's body becomes changed. This is a very frequent early symptom in severe schizophrenia . . . When all ego cathexis is withdrawn from parts of the body, the queerest distortions of self-perception of the body are complained of, or merely described, by the patient . . .' In another section, Federn (1953), describing the distortions of the bodily ego feeling in normal states and dreams, concludes, 'Hence we arrive at the firm conviction that the evidence of the bodily ego boundary must be retained in order that the outer world may remain evident. We possess therefore . . . a permanent evidential feeling of the outer world which originates in the fact that impressions from the outer world pass a bodily ego boundary charged with a particular quality of sensation and bodily ego feeling.' Our observations pointed to a very profound disturbance of bodily ego feeling in our patients. The therapist's stimulation of parts of the patient's face and his verbal reinforcement of the distinction between the patient's body and the external environment would tend to increase bodily awareness thereby strengthening the ego and so lead to the gradual improvement described. The anxiety and aggressive reaction which was the patient's response to the closeness of the therapist could be understood as a fear of fusion. The following description by a patient of Jacobsen's (1954) illustrates the vulnerable feelings experienced by the schizophrenic. ' "Do you know the difference between closeness, likeness, sameness and oneness? Close is close, as with you; when you are like somebody, you are only like the other; sameness—you are the same as the other, but he is still he and you are you; but oneness is not two—it is one, that's horrible—horrible!" She repeated, jumping up in sudden panic, "Don't get too close, get away from the couch, I don't want to be one with you" and she pushed me away very aggressively.'

It has often been reported that physical illness produces an improvement in psychotic conditions. Mayer-Gross (1954) writing on this subject states, 'The influence of acute febrile infections on chronic schizophrenics has for a long time attracted the attention of psychiatrists. During such an illness all the more prominent symptoms, such as stupor, mannerisms, delusional ideas, may disappear and the patient, who was hitherto regarded as being completely demented, may become accessible, show adequate emotions naturally expressed, and take an interest in his surroundings . . . The mechanism of improvement when it occurs is not well understood. There may be some direct influence on the unknown physical disorder underlying the disease. In view of the known tendency to habit function in schizophrenia, the curative effect may be purely psychological. The apparently deteriorated patient may remain inaccessible although the schizophrenic process has come to a standstill. If the bodily disease occurs at that moment, the change of surroundings, the personal attention and the physical suffering may free him from symptoms which become only habit . . . Neither of these suggestions, however, is very satisfying.' We also encountered this phenomenon on several occasions. For example, one day, George Johnson, normally a demented patient, returned to the analytic group after a few days' absence with influenza. He said that he had been talking to Attendant Cairns and that he did not think these meetings did him any good. He spoke for some time in this same vein with unaccustomed clarity and reasonableness. The authors suggest the possibility that the physical illness with the increased bodily sensations leads to increase in the cathexis of the bodily ego with consequent remission of the psychotic process.

An interesting and relevant observation was made by the nurses in the treatment centre. They reported to us that Cathy, our mute catatonic patient already mentioned in this section, did not maintain her improvement throughout the day. Gradually speech and spontaneous movement became less. However, over a period of months they reported that there were days on which she responded to them, spoke freely, and moved about the room. At first neither we nor the nurses could find any explanation for these remissions, until finally it was observed that her episodic improvements coincided with her weekly bath. Again, we are of the opinion that the sensory stimulation awakened had the effect of increasing awareness of the bodily self.

CHAPTER SEVEN

Disturbances in Perception

In Chapter Five we have attempted to illustrate what, in our opinion, is the basic disturbance in schizophrenia—the dissolution of ego boundaries and loss of ego feeling resulting in the patient's unsureness of his own identity and his lack of a clear-cut discrimination between himself and his environment. It is our contention that perceptual disorders typical of schizophrenia can be understood as consequences of this basic disturbance. The capacity for discriminating between oneself and the environment normally varies through a range from the clear-cut awareness of the active waking state on the one hand to the confused state which precedes sleep, the latter being a close approximation to the state of severely disturbed psychotic patients. As the ego boundaries blur and merge with the external environment all perceptual functions are increasingly acted upon by the elements peculiar to primary process thinking. This process which explains the break with reality found in chronic psychotic patients is described by Federn (1953) in the following passage on the results of breakdown of ego boundaries—'On this basis the assumption is made that the schizophrenic loss of reality consists in loss of cathexis of the mental and bodily ego boundary. (Normally.) Whatever is sensed as mere thought is a mental process lying inside the mental and physical ego boundary; whatever is sensed as being real lies outside the ego boundary.'

One result of the weakened ego function and consequent lack of sensory organization is seen in the schizophrenic's susceptibility to environmental stimuli, which he is unable to perceive in their proper order and context. During one session, Jessie was sitting with her face pressed against a therapist, talking rapidly and intently. At the other end of the room another therapist made a remark to a patient: 'You think I only like married ladies.' Without halting in her flow of speech Jessie immediately said, 'Yes, I like married ladies.' A few minutes later another patient addressing the second therapist, said, 'It puts them through a dream.' Again, Jessie's communications with the first therapist contained the apparently irrelevant remark, 'Yes, but you have to wake up.' This incorporation of random stimuli into the patient's stream of talk was very common and explained much of the apparent bizarreness and lack of purpose in the speech content. One is reminded of the resemblance here to the type of egocentric speech Piaget (1932) observed in young children who incorporate random events in the environment into their 'monologues.'

Again, the profound perplexity and uncertainty so often seen in disturbed schizophrenic patients might be viewed as a further extension of the basic uncertainty of their own existence as an integral self. One of the group patients, Emily, in particular, showed this perplexity in all her responses to objects or persons in her environment. The majority of her verbalizations were put forward in a querulous questioning form and she demonstrated a profound uncertainty in identifying objects, places, and persons. For example, in one session she speaks of 'a place *called* the laundry, patients *called* us, a woman *called* her, nurses *called* "hems," a wreck *called* Emily, etc.' While there would seem to be enough residual ego functions to enable her to make some rudimentary discrimination in her perception of external objects, the tenuous and primitive nature of this discrimination is evident in her attachment of crude identifying labels on these objects. This primitive type of discrimination is of course an illustration of the manner of concrete thinking seen in schizophrenia but this subject will be more fully discussed in a later section.

These examples have demonstrated the patient's confusion as to the locus and meaning of sensations and experiences emanating from the external environment. However, the schizophrenic's reduced capacity to experience himself as a separate and distinct entity, with a personal identity, leads also to similar difficulties in locating and organizing perceptions arising from internal stimuli.

One of the patients had a constant facial tic, which culminated in his making a clicking noise with his mouth. Asked about this, he declared it was caused by a bee which had got into his head and was buzzing around. Another female patient perceived sexual sensations as 'little manny beasties biting me here.' This type of reaction to internal sensations comes close to the classical 'kinaesthetic hallucinations' and provides probably the simplest illustration of the disturbed psychotic's inability to perceive his own bodily sensations as part of himself.

Probably the most frequent perceptual disturbances in schizophrenia are auditory hallucinations. In normal psychiatric usage this term describes the condition where the patient 'hears voices' which appear to have their source in the external environment. In a recent article, S. Karagulla (1955) objects to the common tendency to regard these phenomena in such a narrow context and makes an interesting analysis of the range of such perceptual disturbances. 'In schizophrenia the patient is continually troubled by ideas which are presented to him independent of his volition. Some appear to him as though emanating from voices in the external environment. These, the commonly accepted auditory hallucinations, represent in our opinion but one gradation of this experience. The term "auditory hallucinations" cannot be made to cover all the modes of perception of this phenomenon, nor does it sufficiently stress its intricate nature, the intimate relationship which exists between it and the patient's own thought. In some patients those alien ideas appear as "thoughts" differing only slightly in quality from the silent imperceptible flow of normal thinking.' This concept of a gradation of hallucinatory experience would seem to be important in our understanding of the fully developed, bizarre type of hallucinations one finds in chronic schizophrenia. Karagulla's description of the initial stages in the illness, when the ideas merely appear as alien thoughts outside the patient's stream of directed volitional thought, bears a striking resemblance to certain variations of the normal state of consciousness. Fatigue states, day-dreaming, and fever states are a few of the situations where the normal adult experiences the intrusion of non-volitional ideas into his flow of thought. The autonomous nature of the thought processes in free-association could also be regarded as another extension of these phenomena. *In fact it would appear that any situation which involves reduced awareness of the mental and bodily ego, leads to an experience of the thought processes as divorced from the control of the individual, and therefore as alien and externally located.* An illustration of this connection between the awareness of the bodily ego and the occurrence of perceptual disturbances has been provided in an experiment carried out with students in Canada and reported in an article by Hebb (1955). Here the subjects were sealed up in a cubicle for twenty-four hours during which time they merely lay on a bed. Frosted glass goggles, ear plugs, and special suiting were worn to prevent the subject receiving anything but minimal visual, auditory, or tactile perception. Most subjects reported a strange feeling of 'otherness' or 'bodily strangeness' which they found difficulty in describing. One subject said that his mind was 'like a ball of cottonwool' floating in the air above him while others reported that their bodies were 'overlapping in space.' Although detailed description of these experiences is not given, they would seem to have much in common with the state we have been discussing where the boundary between the self and the external world is weakened. But from our point of view the most interesting feature of the experiment lies in the fact that each subject reports a variety of exceptionally vivid auditory and visual hallucinations.

This view, that the psychotic process is essentially dominated by the ego's inability to discriminate between external reality and inner mentality, allows us to comprehend the nature of the bizarre type of hallucinations experienced by the chronic schizophrenic. One patient, Andrew Gray, for example, experienced thoughts of an obscene and sexual nature. These thoughts he described as being produced by a machine which was like 'an old granny blethering away.' The machine would often urge him to masturbate or to carry out other sexual practices. On other occasions he experienced nocturnal images of a similar nature and would again externalize these images—'That machine was showing me pictures last night of Miss M's backside.' He regarded both the form and content of these experiences as being entirely foreign, and complained bitterly about the machine and its 'filthy mind.' Thus the patient's own thoughts, lacking ego feeling and therefore a sense of inner 'belongingness,' are perceived by him as externally located auditory and visual experiences. This type of hallucinatory activity also illustrates the close correspondence between memory and perception already referred to in Chapter Two. This aspect of the memory process will be discussed in a later section dealing with disorders of memory present in schizophrenic patients. It is interesting here to compare these experiences with the 'hallucinations,' reported by Penfield and his co-workers, in the series of experiments involving electrical and cortical stimulation of patients suffering from temporal lobe epilepsy. Similar experiences are reported by patients prior to, or during, actual epileptic convulsions. In the article by Karagulla, to which we have already referred, there occurs the following vivid description given by a temporal lobe patient prior to losing consciousness, '. . . he was aware of all his thoughts transforming themselves into vivid external images. For instance, he thought of fire-crackers and suddenly they were seen in sunset colours . . . in front of his eyes . . . Finally he thought of himself lying on the ground and immediately saw an external pictorial image of himself, described thus: "The way I felt on the ground was the way I looked in the picture but people were not around me. I was in different forms; I thought of something and then I saw it. I thought of myself and then I saw myself the way I was thinking of myself."' One is faced with the suggestion that these seizures, involving, as they do, alterations in consciousness, induce the same disruption in ego boundaries as in the psychotic state with the consequent perceptual distortions which are described. One important difference of course is that the epileptic patient is able to realize *in retrospect* that his experiences are internally motivated, while the chronic schizophrenic is unable to make this check with reality. It is interesting to note that Penfield (1954), speaking of the changes in consciousness occurring in seizures and in response to electrical stimulation, defines consciousness as follows: 'Consciousness, therefore, may be considered as the state of being aware of one's own thought and purposes. The content of one's thought varies greatly from an awareness of sense perception to reflection and meditation. The present purposes may take origin in earlier mental processes or in the thinking of the moment.' There is much correspondence between this definition and our own views on ego feeling.

Having established the point that, in our opinion, the schizophrenic's perceptual disturbances are a necessary consequence of the lack of adequate ego boundaries with the subjective estrangement of ego feeling, we can go on to discuss the development and significance of the delusions observed in the patients studied. While hallucinations are a direct result of the withdrawal of ego cathexis, resulting in the patient's thoughts being experienced as real, we regard the delusion as the patient's attempts to deal with this confusion of reality. We thus agree with Katan (1954) that '. . . the delusion is the result of the attempt to repair the break with reality.' The delusion is the patient's way of coming to terms with his false realities and, to some extent, correlating these with the correct perceptions of the external world. Federn (1953) in fact speaks of the delusion as part of the 'self-healing process of psychosis.' We might look on the delusion as almost a secondary elaboration of the hallucination, indicating as it does the disintegrated ego's attempt to order the ego-alien ideas in accordance with events in the external world.

As already mentioned in Chapter One, the patients who were the subjects of our observations could be roughly divided into two main categories or extremes. One such extreme was the completely disintegrated patient who appeared to live in a permanent world of confusion. Here the ego is fragmented and the resulting picture is of a chaotic lack of integration between the internal and external world. The completely withdrawn catatonic patient we would tend to regard as an end product of this chaotic process where ego cathexis is at a minimum, rendering contact with the external world correspondingly minimal. In the 'demented' type of patient hallucinatory material was abundantly evident, whereas organized delusions were never encountered. The other group of chronic patients were distinctly characterized by a relatively high degree of ego functioning. They retained the ability to converse in non-symbolic terms and were capable of some measure of abstract thought. The manner and degree of residual ego functioning in this type of chronic patient will be discussed in a later section but, for the purposes of the present discussion, it is sufficient to note that it was this type of patient who provided delusional material. The following clinical material taken from these patients provides illustrations of the delusional process at work. It helps us to understand the essentially dynamic adaptive nature of the delusion working as a homeostatic mechanism to define outer reality in accordance with inner mentality.

As already mentioned, Andrew Gray experienced hallucinations of a voice which whispered obscenities in his ear and urged him to masturbate and swear. At other times he experienced visual images, mentioned above, which were again sexual in nature. These experiences were often of a manifestly homosexual type. The genesis of this patient's hallucinations becomes evident when his past history is considered. From his early youth Andrew had participated in a number of incidents with older men involving fellatio and other homosexual stimulation. The beginning of his psychotic breakdown occurred when he was posted by the R.A.F. to a lonely station on the Orkneys where, it can be suggested, the intense pressure of a small closely knit all-male culture proved too strong for his basic homosexual conflicts. The voices and visual images the patient now began to experience represented his own homosexual urges which were unacceptable to the ego, and so lost the ego cathexis necessary to identify them as originating within the psyche. The externalization of his own thought processes, concurrent with the break with objective reality, led to the further adjustment which reunited outer reality and the inner processes that had become the psychotic 'reality.' This adjustment took the form of an unknown individual who tormented him with 'a machine' that communicated to him the oral and visual obscenities so repugnant to his own ego. On occasions he would declare his suspicions that the operator of this 'f——ing machine' was an older man who had first persuaded him to indulge in fellatio. His description of the machine itself being like 'an old granny blethering away' has also significance as the patient was reared for the most part by his rather prim grandmother. The reality adjustive function of this delusion became evident when the patient was faced with interpretations which threatened its existence, when his reaction was to refuse further attendance at the groups.

Once a basic delusion is established the patient indulges in further rationalizations and elaborations to defend the ego's link with reality from all contradictions provided by the objective external world. Thus the original delusion may lead to a progressive number of subsidiary delusions in support of the patient's tenuous hold on reality. This autonomous process was seen clearly in the behaviour of Barbara Thomson in the female group. This patient believed herself to be surrounded by numerous children whom she regarded as her own, addressing each by a different name. She made many stereotyped movements which came to be understood as the various actions involved in feeding and playing with her children. The origin of this basic delusion was never clearly ascertained although it was obviously related to the patient's ambivalent feelings towards her mother and married sister. It soon became clear however that many other delusional beliefs held by the patient were defensive extensions of the primary delusion. Barbara, for example, denied the existence of two sexes and produced long abstract arguments to the effect that each person was bisexual. This further distortion of reality enabled her to be the mother of her phantasy children while still denying that they were the product of any sexual activity on her part. The fact that others declared that they could not see the children was answered by Barbara's assertion that they were so tiny as to be invisible to the casual observer.

A most interesting example of the emergence of a delusion and its relation to past and present reality was provided by a female patient, Mary Bruce. For many years this patient had been a typical example of the aggressive, completely demented chronic patient. She was dishevelled in appearance and of dirty habits, while her speech was so highly symbolic as to be almost incomprehensible. It was noticed that she became most disturbed and violent when approached by any other person and made many references to being interfered with or sexually assaulted. This patient was among those chosen to attend the treatment centre, the function of which will be discussed in detail in Chapter Ten. The patient made a gradual but startling improvement, her aggressive outbursts became less frequent and more comprehensible as responses to frustration in her environment. Within eight months of her attending the centre she no longer appeared to be psychotic. Arrangements were made for her brother to take her home at week-ends. However, several happenings conspired to make her first week-end at home a traumatic experience. A gastric infection which had infected the ward caused Mary to be very sick while at home. More upsetting however was the patient's visit to the grave of her mother who had died while Mary was acutely ill in hospital and so unable to appreciate the reality factors involved in this loss. When Mary returned to hospital after the week-end she was extremely depressed and held an unshakeable delusion that she was pregnant, finally divulging that she felt her brother to be responsible for her condition as they had spent the week-end together at home alone. The influence of the realization of her mother's death, her sickness, and the new relationship with her brother caused by her mother's death were undoubtedly strong motivating factors in the content of her delusion. However, the aspect we wish to stress here is that Mary did not return to her former chaotic state in spite of the traumatic experience involved. Apart from her delusion, her improvement was maintained and her behaviour continued to be reality-orientated and rational. Only when her delusional belief was threatened by interpretations did she show any traces of her previously very disturbed behaviour.

In the treatment centre the patient retained the pregnancy delusion for two months but gradually she expressed less certainty over it until finally she was able to relinquish the belief and speak of it in terms of 'just imagination.' Arrangements were again made for her to begin to live at home. Unfortunately, an administrative error caused the patient to be prevented from going home. Within a few days Mary again became depressed and developed the delusion that she had venereal disease and had infected the nurse in the treatment centre to whom she was deeply attached. Her concern in this case was not for her own condition but for the nurse whom she believed she had infected. This fact alone indicated the more mature and outgoing nature of the ego at this stage, and was taken, in comparison with her previous delusion of pregnancy, to be a more prognostically hopeful sign. When the error was corrected she again improved and the delusion disappeared within a week. This patient has now been fully discharged and is living an energetic symptom-free life at home.

This example draws our attention to the fact that the hallucination or delusion is invariably stimulated by the patient's present experiences. Our observations of hallucinatory activity on the part of patients has led us to believe that such activity is closely related to the patient's present needs and the persons in the environment who may be the means of gratifying these needs. It is often in the activities and emotional responses of persons with whom the patient has an emotional relationship that we find the stimulus to hallucination or delusion. This is demonstrated in the example by Mary's reactions to outside events, but there is ample evidence from the behaviour of patients that outbursts of hallucinatory and delusional activity were invariably 'triggered off' by the actions of significant figures in their environment. Emily often reacted violently to the therapist paying attention to other patients. On these occasions she would stand in the middle of the room looking up at the ceiling and shouting angrily that her hated stepmother was 'Pinching my men and is upstairs in bed f——ing with her husband who doesn't belong to her.' The meaning of this type of disturbance can be traced to the patient's earlier experiences, but fully understood only when its relevance to present events is appreciated.

The vital significance of the role of events and people in the present environment of patients in deciding the content of the psychosis and the form of the behaviour produced is a theme that will be taken up later in Chapter Ten.

CHAPTER EIGHT

Disturbances of Thinking

The disruption of the normal thinking process has long been regarded as a central feature of schizophrenic psychopathology and has been the subject of numerous investigations. It is neither within the scope of this monograph nor cogent to the authors' purpose to attempt an exhaustive appraisal of the literature on schizophrenic thinking. As in previous sections we will discuss the manifestations of disordered thinking from the standpoint of our basic orientation, that the disease process is basically an ego disturbance resulting in a disruption of the boundary between the self and the not-self. Our aim is to understand the factors that produce the chronic schizophrenic patient, in the hope that if they are understood, measures can be taken to help the patient.

With this end in view we have sub-divided this chapter into four sections. The first section illustrates the mechanisms of primary process thought that dominate the productions of the patients studied. We then follow with a discussion of the role of symbolism in the thought processes and the importance of the primary process mechanism in symbol formation. The third section consists of a brief mention of the phenomenon of concrete thinking demonstrated by the patients, and its relation to the similar type of thinking found in children and in cases of brain damage. Finally we refer to the positive aspects of the chronic schizophrenic patient's thinking under the general term 'Synthetic Thinking.' These divisions are of course an artificial abstraction as the processes involved are, as we hope to show, interdependent.

I. PRIMARY PROCESS THOUGHT

In Chapter Five we introduced and developed the theme that the central feature of the schizophrenic disease process is the withdrawal of ego cathexis resulting in loss of self-experience and inadequate differentiation between the self and the environment. This disruption of ego feeling in chronic schizophrenia leads to a weakening of the secondary process thought mechanisms dominant in normal thinking, these being dependent on an adequately functioning ego. This results in the thought process coming increasingly under the control of the primary process mechanisms, the most important of which are condensation and displacement. Although we discuss condensation and displacement separately the distinction is an artificial one for the two are always found together.

(a) *Displacement*

While displacement is usually associated with complex ideational activity it can exist in a primitive form with a much simpler purpose, the gratification of a drive. Studies of early infancy show this clearly. Hoffer (1950), in particular, stresses the relationship between hand and breast in the nursing child. He shows how the child by the process of displacement from the breast learns to suck its hand to reduce tension.

Patients sometimes behave as if they fail to distinguish between objects in their environment and in consequence this leads to the discharge of a drive upon the nearest, rather than the most appropriate, object. For example, during one session David became increasingly irritated with a therapist. He was on the opposite side of the room from the therapist and suddenly kicked Alec who was beside him. When the therapist asked Alec if he had been hurt, David pulled up his own trouser and examined his leg, which he rubbed grunting as though in pain. Examples of this fundamental type of displacement were not very frequent and only occurred in the most disordered type of patient.

The majority of schizophrenic communications and activities

contain many examples of displacement. We noticed that angry patients would direct their attention to the table and push at it furiously after some incident which had evoked their anger against someone in the room. On one occasion a therapist had made a comment about a patient's difficulty with her mother. The patient screamed angrily, ending by rushing at him screaming, 'You're just a filthy old sock.' She stood in front of him, turned away uncertainly, and then rushed over to a corner where a large ornament stood on a pedestal. She took it up, shook it angrily, then set it back shouting at it, 'I'll throw you on the carpet.' This particular vase was the object of a great deal of displaced emotion. For example, one female patient made manifest sexual overtures to one of the therapists. She repeatedly invited him to come upstairs with her, finally turning away and crossing the room slowly to the corner where the vase was standing. She stroked it gently, leaned her cheek against it, and kissed it several times.

These examples of displacement to inanimate objects clearly show an element of purpose. They allowed discharge of feeling and at the same time enabled the patient to avoid a focus of excitation in the environment. A somewhat more complicated instance occurred in the male group. We had been making many comments to a patient, Jim Brown, and pressing him to talk until he appeared quite agitated and distressed. George Johnson, a very artistic person, picked up a piece of paper and made a quick sketch. He described it as follows. 'It is two bears. They are trying to lower a blind man down a well to collect food and drink at the bottom.' This displacement from the immediate situation to the drawing showed George's reaction to the well-meaning attempts on the part of the therapists to force Jim to speak regardless of the anxiety aroused. In this example the mechanism of condensation is as marked as the displacement, and the material is beginning to show a form resembling more closely the finished product of dream work.

As we have already said, displacement is rarely seen as an isolated mechanism. Condensation and other mechanisms are also present, as shown in the following example. A therapist entered the room with a nurse. Emily stared up at the ceiling and began to shout angrily, 'She is standing up there like a nurse. Scram! You are not going to be a nurse. Take any man she wishes and take her body to hell out of here. That fat old bitch up there should scram. She is not a sister. She is looking for trouble. Some man is going to get that bloody brunette into trouble. She does not know what is in store for her. She is going to sleep alone for evermore.' Emily, at that time, had a somewhat tenuous relationship with the therapist in question. Whenever she felt he was paying attention to someone else, she would shout at the ceiling as though she were addressing people upstairs. The content of what she said was derived in part from recollections of the arrival of an obese stepmother at her home. For example, on one occasion the particular therapist, who had been speaking to her, left and crossed over to talk with another patient. Emily at once jumped to her feet and began to shout angrily and obscenely. 'What's that noise? Shut up! It's that bloody fat old bitch in bed f——ing with a man who does not belong to her. She's a stupid fat old bitch and she expects me to bring home a pay-packet to keep her in bed with someone else's man. She's on my name. I'm not going to scrub floors for her.' This memory was invariably recalled and relived whenever the patient's jealousy was aroused and this phenomenon will receive attention later.

(b) *Condensations*

Again when considering the simplest of the condensations shown by these chronic schizophrenic patients, it is important to remember the lack of adequate discrimination between the self and the environment, and the objects contained therein. This confusion of objects in itself is the prototypical condensation. In the example given where David examined his own leg after kicking another patient the two objects are condensed into one.

Similar in nature to these confusions of objects was the constant recurrence of the use of part of some object for the whole object.

Men were referred to as 'socks' and nurses as 'hems' or 'capes,' 'black silk,' or, on a rainy morning, as 'waterproofs.' In our opinion this is a sufficient explanation for these simple condensations, though, as will be illustrated later, similar terse statements represented condensations of very complex type. This type of condensation occurred most frequently in relation to those who were most active in the patients' environment—namely the nurses and doctors, the part-object having some characteristic which attracted the patients' attention, *e.g.*, the bright red border of the nurses' cloak.

The use of the part for the whole would sometimes lead to short statements which condensed an immediate emotional reaction. For example, during the first week of clinical work Emily appeared suspicious. Both therapists, at that time, were smoking pipes. On one occasion when a therapist approached Emily sucking his pipe, she shouted angrily, 'Humph! Stinking government.'

Such examples of condensations were constantly present and it was important to be aware of their nature, as otherwise significant reactions to the staff were not appreciated. Jessie, who disliked the therapist leaving her in order to speak to other patients, on one occasion when he was softly trying to coax a reply from a catatonic patient from whose nose mucus was running commented, 'He's doing slobbery nursing.' At one time a therapist decided to behave in a less permissive way. He attempted to prevent one of the female patients from using the telephone by direct prohibition, and finally by restraining her. The communications of the other patients were replete with condensed references to this incident. One of them said, 'I wonder about this building. All over Scotland there are castles and places where they used to have torture chambers and dungeons to keep people in.' The patient who had been restrained was looking at a magazine with the therapist the following day. She was restless and finally referred to him as 'a policeman reading a Bible straight.'

A change of policy led to one of the authors adopting a new role—that of therapist in a group where he had previously been the observer. He launched himself into the task with enthusiasm. Jessie greeted him with, 'You're a bus with a big bumper,' condensing her view of his enthusiasm with the sexual nature of his interpretations. Later she said, 'You just charge in without looking around.'

2. SYMBOLIC FUNCTIONING

The role of symbol formation in normal and pathological thinking has received detailed study by many investigators operating in many different fields. The resulting concepts are manifold and often contradictory, dependent as they are on the basic orientation of the different investigators. There is even as yet no universally accepted concept as to what constitutes a symbol. We should therefore like to stress that our interest in the development and functioning of symbolic thought is confined to an understanding of the role of symbols in the thinking of chronic schizophrenics.

E. Jones (1916) in his well-known article 'The Theory of Symbolism,' discusses at length the vague broadness of the concept of symbolism in modern usage and differentiates between ideas that are merely 'indirectly represented' and those that are actually symbolized, giving only to the latter the description 'true symbolism.' That this differentiation is not merely of the nature of Piaget's distinction between a sign and a symbol (the sign being related to the thing signified simply by social convention) becomes apparent in Jones's enumeration of the differential characteristics of a 'true symbol'—'representation of unconscious material, constant meaning, independence of individual conditioning factors, evolutionary basis, linguistic connections, and phylogenetic parallels in myths, cults, religion, etc.' Jones makes the further definite statement that 'all symbols represent ideas of the self and the immediate blood relatives, or of the phenomena of birth, love and death.'

While in agreement with this attempt to distinguish between indirect representation and fully developed symbolism, we cannot accept his strict criteria for 'true symbolism' involving a rigid demarcation between the two aspects of symbol formation. Rapaport (1951), while tending to support Jones's classification, is more cautious in his differentiation, suggesting that 'the natural transition between indirect representation and symbolization is a more continuous one . . .' Kubie (1951) is less tentative in his criticism of the rigidity of Jones's criteria, declaring that the distinction between 'indirect representation and symbolism' is to him 'a distinction without an essential difference which may be positively misleading.' Kubie goes on to say, 'It would hardly seem necessary to remind ourselves that there are no such discontinuities in nature as those who put the symbolism of dreams in a category of its own would seem to imply.' Later Kubie also points out that this distinction is not in accordance with Freud's own statement that the idea of the symbol 'cannot be sharply delimited at all times—it mingles with substitution, dramatization, and even approaches allusion.'

In our treatment of symbolic functioning we will regard indirect representation and fully developed symbolism as opposite poles of a continuum, including both as elements of symbol formation. We shall later develop the argument that this continuum represents a primitive thought process analogous to normal rational thought and that the transition from indirect representation to unconscious symbolic thought is causally paralleled by the degree of 'self-awareness' or consciousness of the ego which is present. In brief, we shall try to demonstrate the close correspondence between symbolic thinking and inadequate ego functioning.

We have already referred in the previous section to the vague generalizations and abstractions used by the chronic schizophrenic where a group of objects, people, or ideas are represented by a feature that is common to each element of the group. Emily, it will be remembered, often referred to the nurses as 'capes,' 'hems,' or 'waterproofs,' and to other males as her brothers, to doctors as 'stethoscopes' and to the therapists as 'the government.' Rapaport (1951) suggests that this type of abstraction clearly belongs to the context of normal concept formation, and with this we would agree. The simplest aspect of this can be seen in the thinking of the young child and is appropriately illustrated in the following example described by Werner (1940). A child of four-and-a-half years developed a fear of spiders which soon grew to encompass the spiders' webs. One day the child found a hair stuck on his hand. He screamed in terror, and when his mother was removing the hair, regarded her with amazement asking, 'Didn't the hair bite your finger?' Werner says of this, 'The global quality of biting is related not merely to the spider but to everything characteristic of the spider web. . . . The structure of the percept is homogeneous. It can be described by the familiar phrase—*pars pro toto*—any part has the quality of the whole.' This would appear to be the same primitive perceptual process as demonstrated by Emily's reference to nurses as 'capes,' 'hems' or 'waterproofs' depending on the article worn at the time. Although appearing to generalize about a group of people, Emily was in fact only using a sensory impression common to the group. This type of indirect representation appears to have no emotional determinant, being dependent on a primitive form of sensory perception. Other representations, such as Emily's references to other men as her brothers and to the therapists as 'the government,' were however more frequently made and, in our opinion, contain an emotional significance not present in the simple *pars pro toto* examples. Interesting comparisons can be found in ethological studies. In recent years observers have demonstrated that the behavioural response of animals to objects is governed by certain factors which Werner refers to as 'dominant signals' and Lorenz and Tinbergen as 'sign stimuli.' Thus a spider responds not to a fly in its web but to a specific vibration which can actually be determined. Again, Lorenz has shown that birds respond to the concept of a hawk on the basis of a shape with a determinable relationship between the length of head and neck as compared with the body. Thus the essence of a fly to a spider is a certain vibration and the essence of 'hawkness' to the bird is a certain size ratio. Moving upwards in the evolutionary scale to the observation of children, one is reminded of the similarity in the young child who, when asked to draw a man, draws a head and legs, resisting all suggestions of addition. The child in fact draws his emotional essence of the concept of 'man,' and this phenomenon can be observed in many children's drawings. Werner, whose concept of physiognomic perception is similar to this process, quotes a child of four-and-a-half years referring to a camera tripod as 'proud' when it stood vertically, and 'sad' when it leaned at a precarious angle. Now let us return to the schizophrenic adult patient. In his footnote to Bleuler's (1912) reference to Wernicke's patient responding to his attendant as his sister, Rapaport declares, 'Something about the attendant (for example, friendliness or cruelty) led to his being physiognomically subsumed as "friendly" or "cruel" in the same relative category in which the patient's sister was an outstanding object.' It is a similar process that we regard as being the basis of Emily's representation of certain men as her brothers and of the therapists and other medical staff as 'the government.' Perhaps a clearer example of this was provided by Barbara Thomson who, when the observer newly joined the group as a therapist, greeted him as a woman. The following day she explained that the therapist had been 'speaking softly and timidly like my sister.' He had indeed been aware of his timidity and lowered voice due to his inexperience and uneasiness in entering the group for the first time. Arieti (1948 and 1955), who has also made an extensive study of schizophrenic thought disorder, forms the concept of 'paralogic' thinking introduced by Van Domarus to the effect that the schizophrenic 'accepts identity on the basis of identical predicates.' Thus the soft voice and timid manner in the example just quoted is a common predicate identifying the therapist with the patient's sister. Missing in this concept of paralogic thinking is the emotional significance of the selection of a particular identifying characteristic. The quietness of voice and timidity might, in Barbara's case, have had a specific emotional meaning in the patient's relation to her sister. The possible significance of an emotional factor in determining the use of a symbol is also illustrated by the following example.

One of Emily's names for nurses was 'ruffs.' These were the soft white cuffs which were used to cover the end of the sleeves when they were rolled up. It was observed that she only used this particular word for the nurses when she was annoyed with them. One day the nurse spoke to one of us at the door to let us know about an incident which had occurred before they left the ward. Although the patients were not close enough to hear the conversation, they were able to observe this event. When the session began Emily was irritable. She gestured to the nurse, 'Ruffles gets all the money.' One of the therapists said, 'You knew someone before who wore ruffs.' Emily sprang to her feet—'She has a big John. She can go to that. Every one of her sons can go to work.' Emily's stepmother had in fact worn ruffs at her housework, and this specific meaning was the determinant of its use in a setting of hostility and jealousy to the nurses.

The durability of this and other symbols was, in our opinion, dependent on the extreme emotional significance to the patient of the experience signified by the symbol. In some cases the patient's emotional relationship maintained a durable constellation of symbols with a constant theme reflecting the emotional basis. Jessie Brown used to refer to one of the therapists as a wizard, and many of her symbols for him were derived from this source. On one occasion, when he had been stroking another patient's cheek and that patient had been smiling and speaking to him, she said, 'Come over here and bring your lump of magic with you.' On another occasion, when he had spent more time than usual going round talking to the others, she referred to him as 'Claverhouse going round slavering.' The readers familiar with Scottish myth and history will recall that the Jacobite leader Graham of Claverhouse was reputed by his Covenanter enemies to lead a life of debauchery. They further considered him a wizard and when he was killed at the Battle of Killiecrankie there was a legend that a Covenanter marksman had shot him with a silver bullet—the traditional way of killing wizards. From this central idea—that the therapist was a wizard—sprang a large number of symbols and symbolic communications. The patient used to say of him that he was 'doing tricks,' 'casting a spell' over the patients. She used to threaten him with a 'silver bullet' or a 'silver cannon.' This particular constellation of symbols was quite a constant feature throughout a year of work, in which she maintained a constant relationship with this therapist.

At the beginning of this discourse we referred to Rapaport's assertion that many of the indirect representations that we see in schizophrenia can be categorized as concept formation. In our examples we have tried to show that schizophrenic symbolic thinking does contain an element of logic and in some ways resembles normal conceptual thinking. This point has been well expanded by Piaget (1951) in his treatment of symbolism. 'Condensation and displacement represent here almost functional equivalents of generalization and abstraction—the processes of logical conceptual thought. Condensation involves giving a common meaning to a number of distinct objects. It expresses the assimilation of different situations and is thus akin to generalization. In the same way there can be no condensation without effective displacement, so displacement corresponds to abstraction on the cognitive level. One can say then that unconscious symbolic thought is an extension of normal thinking. . . .' Bleuler (1912), too, has noted that condensation is a variety of concept formation and thus a primitive form of conceptualization.

Before we attempt to make our last point, on the connection between symbol formation and ego disturbance, we should like to refer to an important factor that may be overlooked in our attempts to understand the meanings of symbolic communications. Our recognition of the fact that emotional relationships are the vital factor motivating and producing the symbolic representations must not lead us to lose sight of the role played in the formation of symbols by sometimes quite trivial day-to-day events. For example, one patient frequently used space-ships and space-stations as symbols. It was discovered that this was based on a daily adventure of 'Jeff Hawke,' a character in a strip cartoon. On one occasion, Johnson sat watching and listening for a quarter of an hour while the therapists were talking with other patients. Finally he remarked, 'I see that the Egyptian Prime Minister has not been invited to the meeting of Asiatic Prime Ministers in Ceylon.' He seemed to be conveying his sense of isolation by this reference to news which was in the headlines.

Early in this section we postulated that indirect representation and symbolic thought functioning are opposite poles of a single continuum. The steps in the gradation from one to the other, we will now argue, are dependent on the level of ego functioning that is present. Jones (1916) held that 'true symbolism' was sufficiently explained as a representation of unconscious material and of repressed affect. We believe that a fuller explanation is obtained by taking into account the ego boundary disturbance which is the basis of all schizophrenic disorders. In this aim we enlist the aid of two other investigators of symbolic thought who drew similar conclusions although approaching the problem from different views and by different methods.

Silberer (1912) conducted an exhaustive introspective analysis of symbol formation occurring in the hypnagogic state. He was able to demonstrate that states of fatigue tend to facilitate the representation of thoughts as symbols. He postulated that the basis of symbolism was 'an apperceptive insufficiency of the ego,' the greater this insufficiency, the greater the degree of the subject's unawareness of the meaning of the symbols. Jones objected to this causal linking of symbolism with 'apperceptive insufficiency,' declaring it to be comparable with attempting to explain slips of the tongue as resulting from fatigue. He accused Silberer of oversimplifying the process of symbol formation by ignoring the repressed unconscious affect lying behind the conscious symbol. Silberer's conclusions are however supported by Fenichel (1945), who attempted to reconcile the two divergent views. He pointed out that although symbolic thinking may occur in adults where the purpose is the distortion of a repressed idea, it could also occur 'not only where distortions have to be made but also in states of fatigue, sleep, psychosis, and generally in early childhood, that is, in all states where archaic ego characteristics are in the foreground.' Later Fenichel explained his differentiation of the origin of symbolism. 'However, archaic symbolism as a part of prelogical thinking and distortion by means of representing a repressed idea through a conscious symbol are not the same. Whereas in distortion the idea of penis is avoided through disguising it by the idea of snake, in prelogical thinking penis and snake are one and the same; that is they are perceived by a common conception.' Silberer's concept of 'apperceptive insufficiency of the ego,' of course, closely corresponds to the disturbance of ego boundaries which we have seen to be present in schizophrenia.

Piaget (1951) approaches the problem of symbolism from the standpoint of his study of thinking in young children with special reference to the dream state. However, his conclusions have much in common with Silberer's and lend themselves to excellent adaptation in explaining the development of symbolism in schizophrenic thought. Pin-pointing the key factor which accounts for the subject's inability to comprehend his own symbolism, Piaget declares, 'The unconscious character of the symbol can be explained by the complete egocentrism of dreams and of repressed tendencies. In a state of radical egocentrism there is a complete lack of differentiation between the ego and the external world, and consequently a state of non-consciousness of the ego. The origin of the unconscious symbol is to be found in the suppression of consciousness of the ego by complete absorption in, and identification with the external world . . .' Later Piaget points out that the semi-conscious state of the dreamer is comparable to 'the state of complete egocentrism characteristic of the baby's consciousness' as in each case 'there is a complete lack of differentiation between the ego and the external world.' We would only add that this state is also comparable with that which we have observed to be present in the chronic schizophrenic. Thus we need not invoke repression to explain symbolism in chronic schizophrenia if we assume an egocentrism in which there is no differentiation between ego and external world, and therefore no capacity for reflective thinking through which the subject could comprehend his own symbolism. Nevertheless, it is legitimate for the observer to see meaning in terms of unconscious process.

Finally, in illustration of this explanation of the unconscious nature of symbol formation, let us consider a few examples of more complex symbolic communications occurring in the group of chronic schizophrenics. It is hardly necessary to add that this kind of symbolic communications occurred most frequently with our most demented patients who demonstrated the most profound ego disturbance and the poorest capacity for investing their own thought processes with the cathexes necessary for identifying them as part of their own ego.

Earlier we quoted an example where George Johnson conveyed his feelings of rejection and isolation in the group by a reference to the Egyptian Prime Minister not being invited to the meeting of Asiatic Prime Ministers. Denied ego accommodation the experience is represented symbolically in a condensed, displaced form, much as it might be represented in a dream where again consciousness of the ego is absent.

Another patient, Myra Green, described her change of attitude to the two therapists, from one of terrified withdrawal to spontaneous contact, as follows, 'I was frightened of the two umbrellas in case their handles damaged me, so I stayed out in the rain. Now, I'm not frightened any more and I shelter under the umbrellas.'

Here, again, the patient's ambivalent feelings of the therapists as protectors and as sexually dangerous objects is denied ego investment and represented symbolically.

3. CONCRETE THINKING

The concrete nature of the schizophrenic thought process seems at first sight difficult to reconcile with the predominance of symbolic thinking in schizophrenia but, in fact, concrete thought and symbolism are closely related and indeed are in many respects identical. We have argued that symbolic thought is a primitive analogy of normal, rational conceptual thinking by the secondary processes, and that the basis of symbol formation is the state of 'non-consciousness of the ego' (Piaget, 1951), with consequent lack of differentiation between the inner and outer world. It is our opinion that the concreteness of thought apparent in schizophrenia is but another manifestation of this basic ego weakness.

Much has been written on the concreteness of the thought processes expressed by the schizophrenic. Some investigators, Cameron (1939), Vigotsky (1934), Kasanin (1944), *et al.*, have, on the basis of cognitive testing, concluded that the schizophrenic is unable to form the abstractions necessary for normal thinking in much the same manner in which the patient with organic brain defect is unable to deal with abstractions. Others, such as Piaget (1932), studying the development of the thought processes in children, have pointed to the correspondence between the essentially concrete manner of thinking demonstrated by the young child and the thought processes demonstrated by the psychotic. Concrete thinking in children is most prevalent during the first three to four years of life when the discriminating processes between the individual and the environment are still developing. In children in whom this process is halted (autistic children) we find that the manner of thinking is almost entirely concrete in nature. Beata Rank (1949), who has carried out an intensive study of these autistic children, concludes that '. . . such a child was raised in an emotional climate which was not favourable for the development of a clear-cut distinction between the self and the outside world, thus crippling the capacity for identification with the mother . . . and thereby interfering with the development of both a unified personality and the reality principle.'

As mentioned in a previous section, Goldstein (1939), after an extensive study of the behaviour of patients suffering from organic brain damage, concluded that the concreteness of thought so typical of these patients is fundamentally based on their inability to 'experience the world as apart from him' and to 'experience the self as an object akin to other objects.'

Accepting this evidence, we are faced with the general conclusion that in any case where there is inadequate differentiation between the ego and the external environment, the thought processes will be increasingly concrete in nature. In the cases studied in our groups, it was those patients who showed most clearly a pronounced lack of ego differentiation whose thinking was most concrete. To think abstractly one must be able to discriminate clearly between the idea of an object as a real one and as a representation for thinking. It is this discrimination that our patients with a gross disturbance of ego boundaries are unable to make. Jessie Brown, for instance, once became mute, and when pressed about this finally declared, 'The words will be down in ink and I'll never get them back.' This was a reference to the observer who was taking verbatim notes. On another occasion the observer, now functioning within the group as a therapist, approached Jessie. She said, 'If you want to get to know me look in your little black book because you have me there.' One is reminded of Freud's patient (1913) who refused to write her name or show her handwriting at all for fear that in doing so she might lose something of herself. Similarly, Piaget has shown how children frequently believe that their thoughts are material, that others can touch or see their thoughts, and that it is possible for others to take their thoughts away.

Another patient in the refractory ward who usually behaved in a rather prim manner suddenly began to scream obscenities at other patients. When asked why she was swearing, she said, 'I'm throwing them back at them.' On one occasion in the female group, Emily was sitting beside Jessie swearing obscenely. Finally Jessie wrapped her scarf round her face saying, 'I am surrounded by filth. The scarf will help me from becoming dirty.'

The patient's weakened sense of his own identity and the concrete manner of his thinking are again evident in the significance and importance the schizophrenic attaches to his name. On some occasions Emily declared she had no name, and on others she would describe herself as Emily McPhie (her family doctor's surname), Mrs. I-Can-Wait, and by other transient identifying titles. Standing out from her usual uncertainty was her constant conviction that her name was not Emily Smith. During the sessions it gradually emerged that Emily was referring to the marriage of her hated stepmother to her father. 'Her name is Smith. That big bitch from S—— took my name away.' Another patient in the male group, George Johnson, made the following concrete reference when he was questioned about his life prior to his illness. 'An atom bomb fell on me and I lost my identity . . . Jackie Coogan, The Kid, died that night of 2nd October, 1937.' This indeed was the exact date on which the patient became acutely psychotic and he was admitted to hospital the following morning.

Let us attempt to summarize our views on the concrete thinking of schizophrenics on the basis of the material already presented. We have argued that the ability to think abstractly is based on the capacity of the individual to make an adequate, clear-cut discrimination between himself, the external world, and the objects therein. Any factor that decreases this ability leads directly to an increasingly concrete style of thought. On the basis of our observations of schizophrenics, we have concluded that a dissolution of ego boundaries is the basic disturbance that leads to, and colours, all other aspects of the disease process.

Thus, the greater the degree of ego disturbance, the more the patient will demonstrate a concrete attitude in his thinking. This, of course, is merely a further extension of the known fact that concrete thinking, as revealed by cognitive tests, is most evident in the more demented type of schizophrenic. Whatever capacity for abstract thinking remains is governed, not by secondary process factors as in normal thinking, but by primary process factors, notably condensation, displacement, and the patient's individual symbolic values. The more intact the ego function, the more the quality of thinking will approach rational normal thinking. This question of the more positive side of schizophrenic thinking controlled by the residual ego will be elaborated in the following section.

4. SYNTHETIC THINKING

Throughout our discourse on schizophrenic thinking we have

been concerned with its primary process manifestations, which are a result of the disruption of ego boundaries and the consequent break with reality. Although emphasizing this aspect of the schizophrenic thought process we have stressed that, even in the most chronic patient, there is seldom, if ever, complete absence of ego. Under the present heading we would like to comment briefly on the ego functions that remain available to the schizophrenic patient, functions which, from time to time, forcefully remind us that reality is never completely lost, even in the most bizarre demented patient. Federn (1953), although dealing mainly with the loss of ego cathexes, draws attention to the residual ego function operating in the psychotic. 'However in every psychotic . . . some of the ego boundaries remain occupied with realities and with external relationships. . . . In verbal utterances of whatever sort, sometimes the secondary normal process, and sometimes the primary psychotic process may prevail. Most patients use largely the secondary mechanisms, reporting, and keen observations, and correct judgments, but then suddenly employing primary mechanisms, with resulting absurd combinations.' Katan (1954), too, speaks of the 'non-psychotic layer' in schizophrenia which 'increases and decreases in size continually.'

As already mentioned, one can find two broad clinical categories among chronic patients. On the one hand, we have the so-called 'demented' patients—the typical inhabitants of the mental hospital refractory ward. On the other hand, there are those patients who do not 'deteriorate' in habit, maintain a constructive interest in the environment, and on casual contact show little evidence of illness. With these latter, more preserved patients most of their thinking is of a rational, coherent secondary process nature. One finds oneself involved in long, rather superficial talks which show a keen appraisal of the situation and a fairly high order of abstract thought. One such chronic patient, for example, would speak at great length of her previous employment in the civil service and her activities as a staff representative. At times a patient's appraisal of the situation can be uncomfortably keen. At one stage of the male group there was a general demand for something to drink and the authors supplied fruit drinks to those who wished it. Andrew Gray surveyed this scene with distaste, finally remarking, 'Treatment! This place is more like Fusco's: a bloody lemonade and ice-cream shop.' This type of reality-orientated thinking was not however confined to the more preserved chronic patient. From time to time the more chaotic and demented patient would interrupt a flow of primary process material with a remark which would demonstrate the acuity and accuracy of the residual ego function still in operation. On one occasion, Andrew had been speaking of an experience involving fellatio which he had had in the Air Force. David, a very demented patient, was behaving in a restless and disturbed manner, making sucking noises with his mouth. A therapist asked him if he were upset because of remembering some similar experience. David replied, 'That's a horrible thing to say to a man.' It is difficult to convey to the reader the startling incongruity of such a remark coming from a very disturbed man like David who had not previously produced one intelligible statement in several months of work. On another occasion when a discussion of incestuous drives was being held, and David was asked whether he too had experienced such feelings, he replied, 'That's a dreadful accusation to make.' A somewhat similar example is illustrated from the following remark by a female patient. Emily was upset by lack of attention from the therapists. She cursed and gesticulated at the ceiling, speaking as usual of 'The fat old woman who was f——ing in bed.' One of the therapists asked, 'Why do you speak so much about f——ing?' Emily looked shocked and said, 'I'm a woman. Don't use swear words in my presence. You're no doctor to speak like that.' As already mentioned one of the authors, who had acted as observer in the group, became a therapist. On the first occasion when he did this, the first patient he approached was Jessie Brown. Before he spoke, she stopped muttering, looked at him and said, 'It must be a great relief to get away from scribbling in a little black book.' These remarks were, in the case of the demented patient, isolated statements in a veritable sea of incoherent primary process verbalizations.

It was observed however that, as the therapist increased his efforts to communicate with the demented patient, the patient's speech in turn took on more and more coherence and the examples of cogent rational remarks made by the patient became more frequent. For some time we explained this phenomenon on the grounds of the therapist's increasing familiarity with the form of the patient's primary process, thus inferring that it was not a matter of the patient becoming more coherent, but of the therapist obtaining a better understanding of the incoherent primary process material. While there is an element of truth in this explanation, we became increasingly convinced that the patient-therapist communications were also resulting in a change in the form of the patient's verbalizations in the direction of increased lucidity and reality adaptations. One might visualize this as a gradual widening of the ego boundary. This view gains support from Rapaport's (1951) statements on the importance of communication itself in the psychic life of the individual. 'Communication enriches the store of experiences and thereby counteracts ego limitation. . . . The enrichment by experiences originating in the course of communication, in external perceptions and introspective observations—furthers the differentiation of ego interests. . . . Communication enhances the "synthetic function of the ego."' In other words, we might regard communication here as a verbal therapeutic parallel to physical contact, the former increasing awareness of the mental ego as does the latter of the bodily ego.

Thus far we have merely described the presence of normal rational secondary process thought which is seen to be present even in the most demented patient, although, of course, there is an inverse relation between the degree of dementia or reality break and the degree of secondary process thought available.

We would now like to discuss a more interesting manifestation of ego function in the thought processes. We refer here to the ego's function in unifying and elaborating the primary process material in accordance with the reality principle. In Chapter 6 of the *Interpretation of Dreams* (1900), Freud mentions this process as the fourth factor in dream formation, attributing it, however, to the ego which maintains its censoring role even in sleep. Freud names this process 'secondary revision' (1955 translation), stating of it, 'Only in the most extreme cases does the psychic function in dream-formation which we are now considering rise to original creation; whenever possible it makes use of anything appropriate that it can find in the dream material. What distinguishes this part of the dream work, and also betrays it, is this tendency. This function proceeds in a manner which the poet maliciously attributes to the philosopher: with its rags and tatters it stops up the breaches in the structure of the dream. The result of its efforts is that the dream loses the appearance of absurdity and incoherence and approaches the pattern of an intelligible experience.' A similar unifying activity of the ego in waking life is described by Nunberg (1931) who introduces the term 'Synthetic function of the ego.' He points out that the ego will not tolerate contradictions within it. He states, 'Where repression has been most unsuccessful, as for instance, in schizophrenic disturbances in which the repressed material manages to gain direct access to consciousness, rationalization is most plainly in evidence. Here things that are wholly irrelevant to one another are quite uncritically brought into causal relation, because, as I have already said, the ego has a tendency to unify and connect, and is obviously no longer able to tolerate excessive contradictions. But if the ego has undergone complete disintegration, as a rule it no longer even essays the secondary elaboration of unconscious wishes and phantasies, or else if the attempt is made, it is so clumsy that the meaning of the unconscious material is scarcely distorted at all and can be immediately recognized.'

This type of secondary elaboration (the term 'secondary elaboration' is used here in distinction to the parallel process occurring in dreaming for which the term 'secondary revision' is used) of primary process ideas was most apparent in our chronic patients. The following example given by a female patient is typical of this type of production. It will be recalled that in examples given earlier it was shown how the patients, through confusion of themselves with others, frequently were unsure of their sex. This phenomenon occurred particularly in relation to staff members. On one occasion, when the patient had been speaking in a confused and perplexed way on this subject, she said suddenly and quite clearly, 'There are no differences in sex. The difference is only individual. There was a time in the history of mankind when all people were the same and they have evolved differently—each one unique.' The confusion of identity remains clear despite the elaboration by the secondary process activity. This form of elaboration was common in the type of day-to-day verbalization given by the more preserved patients. When finally these patients did cautiously begin to divulge more about their illness, they gave detailed accounts of delusional beliefs of a highly complex and structured nature. Nunberg (1931), writing on this subject, states, '. . . with the total disintegration of the personality the ego's synthetic function fails altogether. When, on the one hand, its stability is most gravely threatened but it yet retains a certain measure of constructive energy (as in the paranoid forms of schizophrenia), its synthetic operations are immeasurably extended . . .' We have already discussed the development and function of delusions earlier in this chapter. It was then suggested that delusion formation can be viewed as a further secondary elaboration of the hallucination, which is itself a result of the breakdown of ego boundaries. The delusion is then seen as another aspect of the synthetic function of the ego, the synthesis aimed at being that between inner and outer reality.

It will be remembered that in discussing symbolic thought we defined it as a primitive extension of the normal thought process, condensation and displacement fulfilling the functions which abstraction and generalization play in normal thinking. Our view here is similar in that the process of secondary elaboration of primary material is again a prototype of the fully developed synthetic ego function prominent in normal thinking. That Freud also visualized such a continuum linking the two thought processes is evident in his comment, 'The following consideration makes it seem very probable that this psychic functioning, which undertakes the so-called secondary revision of the dream content, is identical with the work of our waking thought. Our waking thought behaves towards any given perceptual material precisely as the function in question behaves towards the dream content. It is natural to our waking thought to create order in such material, to construct relations, and to subject it to the requirement of an intelligible coherence.'

As we have already stressed, the appearance of secondary process material was seen not only in the more preserved delusional patient but also, to a lesser extent, in the more demented patient. These occasional interjections of normal reality-orientated thought into a stream of primary material were startling in their occurrences in a patient who superficially appeared to have no link with reality. Of a more startling nature however were the occasions when the demented psychotic was seen for a brief moment to stand outside and observe the psychosis. By this we refer to remarks by patients demonstrating their ability to be aware of their own chaotic state while still a part of this chaos. On one occasion when Jessie had been annoyed by one of the authors who had spoken to another patient in the ward and not to her, she covered her eyes and refused to speak to him. She finally took her hands away from her eyes and began to talk, eventually saying, 'It is better to be mad, the mad don't see.' On other occasions she would say, 'I'm just simple' or 'I'm mad.' A male patient had been speaking to the therapist for a few days. Everything he said was couched in a totally bizarre incoherent form. For the most part the therapist had been a listener. Suddenly the patient declared, 'I'm in a bit of a mess, sir; I'm just a shambles; I have nothing. I need some help to get away from this rubbish.' His speech following this remark immediately relapsed into incoherence. This type of awareness reminds one of Freud's account of dream thought and the experience of 'But it's only a dream.' Such insight is of course an ego activity and is specifically dependent on one aspect of the ego to which we have continually made reference, *i.e.*, the ability to be aware of one's own thought process and feelings. Rapaport (1951), speaking of the absence of this ability in diffuse states of consciousness, declares, 'These states of consciousness in which thought formations of the primary process type abound are as a rule characterized by a limitation or absence of reflective awareness. Drive action and drive cathected ideas (hallucinations, delusions) usually occur unaccompanied by reflective awareness; however, in borderline schizophrenic states, delusions may be accompanied by some such awareness, and it can be present even in dreams: "This is just a dream." On the other end of the continuum, there are dreams which are experienced as full reality. The average run of dreams however has neither of these qualities clearly, and is characterized by a playfully unexplicit awareness, singularly the dream's own.'

As we regard the absence of reflective awareness to be one of the chief aspects of the schizophrenic disease process, we must regard any appearance of such awareness in our chronic patients as a therapeutically hopeful sign, signifying, as it does, that the ego is momentarily clear-cut and stable.

Among the other aspects of ego functioning, not already covered in our discussion of secondary elaboration and synthetic thinking, there is one which seems worthy of mention as we have found it to be a useful prognostic guide during treatment of the chronic schizophrenic. We refer now to the ego's function of providing defences. It will be recollected that in our discussion of the primary process mechanisms, earlier in this chapter, a description was given of the type of displacements which were abundant in their occurrence in the patient's behaviour. In the examples given of displacement, it is evident that they contain an element of purpose as distinct from the primitive 'displacements,' which are explained by the weakened ego's lack of discrimination of external objects. Emily Smith's displacement of threats and abuse on to a vase, instead of directing the aggression towards the therapist, can be seen to involve some degree of ego-directed activity. There is a definite distinction to be made between this type of activity and that of delusion formation and other devices by which the schizophrenic maintains some measure of reality contact. Both are ego activities and both are defensive in function. However, while the type of displacement illustrated is used as a defence allowing the ego to cope with external reality, the delusion operates as a defence to distort outer reality and prevent the remnants of the ego from being overpowered by the primary process material. Emily's behaviour, in fact, differs only in degree from the defences shown by the psychoneurotic patient. Such purposeful ego activity is, however, at a minimum in the chronic psychotic patient, where the need to produce manœuvres in defence of the ego does not often arise owing to the lack of an ego to defend. It is therefore of interest to observe that such defensive mechanisms became increasingly apparent in the behaviour of patients attending the treatment centre. One very demented patient had originally reacted to frustrating situations with outbursts of undirected rage, undirected in the sense that the recipient might be the nurse, another patient, or even a window, table, etc. If the object of her rage was in her immediate vicinity, this person might be attacked, but more often it was the nearest person or object that received the onslaught. Gradually this patient formed a positive relationship with the nurse in the centre and her outbursts now took on a more purposeful form. When this nurse did something which upset the patient she reacted aggressively as before, but the object of attack was now another patient in the centre to whom the nurse had often shown attention. Other patients showed abundant examples of the same type of ego-directed displacement of affect. In short, under the influence of the ego-building forces affecting the patient within the treatment centre, the patient's primary affects were seen to be increasingly under the control of a gradually developing ego.

CHAPTER NINE

Disturbances of Memory

In discussing memory disturbances in schizophrenia we must again first draw attention to the artificiality of the distinction we have made between disturbances of perception, thinking, and memory, processes which are not isolated entities but are dynamically interrelated in the living organism.

Most psychiatric textbooks, from Bleuler (1911) to Mayer-Gross (1954), have regarded memory disturbances as non-apparent in the schizophrenic symptomatology. Bleuler (1911), for example, discussing the process of remembering in schizophrenia, has this to say, 'Memory as such does not suffer in this disorder. Patients reproduce experiences they had before and after the onset of the illness as well as any normal person. In fact, they often recall the latter much better, since their minds register everything with the acuity of a camera . . .' In approaching this aspect of pathological behaviour we would agree with Rapaport's comment (1951) that '. . . the criterion of memory disorder is not whether there is retention but whether retained memories are available when necessary and appropriate.' It is inappropriateness of recall that constitutes the form of memory disturbance which we have observed in our chronic schizophrenics. Certainly some of the most demented patients showed at times an inability to attend to and perceive external events. However, all the patients showed a quite normal capacity in their retention and recall of experiences previously perceived. It was in the temporal sequence of the experiences recalled and their appropriateness to the present situation that the distortions were clearly apparent.

During one period of the female group Emily Smith had been receiving a great deal of attention from one of the therapists. Later the therapist's attention was taken up by other patients in the group and Emily sat in silence for several days. Finally she declared, 'I work in a factory. It is a laundry in Burnside Place. My boss is an old man and his name is John Neilson. I am unemployed this morning. What is going to happen when I leave this laundry?' For some time after this incident Emily repeatedly referred to the hospital as a laundry and to the therapist as 'John Neilson.' A male patient, David Black, showed a temporal distortion in references to experiences with his grandmother, whom he had not seen for over twenty years, whereas the incidents were subjectively recalled as recent events. Betty Jones occasionally spoke in a bizarre manner of chloroform, operating tables, scalpels, and other objects related to her past experiences as a nurse. Again the recall of these experiences was exact, but the patient temporally located them in the present or recent past. At other times recent events were correctly recalled but as temporally remote. Barbara Thomson spoke of meeting one of the therapists when she had first become ill seven years before. Her recall of their meeting and what had been said was correct, but the event had in fact occurred only ten days previously. Accompanying these temporal distortions the patients frequently produced detailed memories which were related as if they had been experienced by another person. For example, on one occasion Emily, on being addressed by her name, said to a therapist, 'I knew a girl called Emily Smith. She worked in a laundry office and she used to be sent round to the Post Office in the mornings for stamps.' At other times memories were produced clearly, but with an accompanying display of perplexity, as the patient tried to identify the 'character' in the memory schema, who was in fact herself.

This type of memory disturbance, which entails an objective temporal distortion and a subjective lack of 'belongingness' to the patient, is again in our opinion a further extension of the basic incapacity, the dissolution of ego boundaries with the resultant loss of self-experience. Federn, in speaking of the disturbance of memory exhibited in the early psychotic patient, declares, 'The memories enter the conscious rapidly and correctly and they are also clearly differentiated, but yet they enter . . . in a remarkably "unegolike" manner.' This description is equally applicable to the type of recall discussed which occurred in our chronic psychotics. It is not so much that the memory process itself is disturbed, but that the experience recalled is no longer invested with the ego cathexes necessary for its subjective acceptance as an ego experience. Remembering our definition of ego feeling as an objectively recognizable and subjectively perceived feeling representing 'the continuity of the person in respect to time, space, and causality,' we can understand the apparently inappropriate mode of recall demonstrated by these patients. Let us again refer to Federn's remarks (1953) on the feeling of 'estrangement' which represents the beginnings of the loss of ego cathexes and characterizes the initial psychotic stage. 'Insufficient continuity manifests itself in the inaccurate feeling for time, past, present and future, the passing of the moment is also vague. A state of mind or an event cannot be differentiated as permanent or as lasting only for a moment. . . . With this vagueness comes uncertainty as to the historical sequence of memories, frequently with a clouded feeling as to whether another person may not have been the actor.' *Our view of this aspect of memory distortion in schizophrenia might then be summarized by saying that these disturbances are merely the temporal aspect of the patient's reduced capacity to experience himself as a continuous person with enduring feelings and experiences.*

Another important aspect of the memory disturbance demonstrated by these patients became apparent during our observation of the type of hallucinatory material that they produced. Andrew Gray, for example, declared that he could not read a magazine because 'that machine is flashing in front of my eyes, showing me pictures of girls I knew when I was sixteen. Now it is showing me pictures of myself in the Royal Air Force and of things I was doing there.' Cathy, a patient in the female group, described the beginning of her illness thus: 'I was not ill. I was mixed up. It was the picture. I went to the pictures, and when I got home I kept seeing the picture. I saw it when I was in bed. It was about a man and a woman doing things—a love picture. The man and woman were someone I knew. The woman looked like me but I can't remember the man's name.' In this instance later statements suggested that the man in the 'picture' was a past boyfriend of Cathy's.

The point we would wish to make regarding this type of hallucination is that it appeared that the content was a direct memory which was being reactivated and appearing as a perception. In the second example given here Cathy again demonstrates the vague 'unegolike' quality of the memory image.

In attempting to understand the mechanism behind these memories being recalled as perceptions we would refer the reader to Chapter Two where the Freudian conceptions of the mind, or the mental apparatus, were set out in detail. It will be remembered that Freud (1900) explained the visual vividness of the dream state as a retrograde movement of the mental energy in the mental apparatus. The excitation normally discharged at the motor end of the apparatus is now reversed and discharged in the form of perceptual images at the perceptual end. Freud further postulated the hallucinatory activity of the infant as a re-experiencing of an earlier perception in the same fashion as the dream image is produced, both resulting from the inadequate state of the ego and the lack of any clear-cut discrimination between the self and the not-self. The schizophrenic patient can be compared both to the infant and to the dreamer in that he too has a weakened sense of ego feeling and a reduced capacity for self-experience. His needs are gratified by the reactivation of a memory image as a perception, as is the infant's need for the mother's breast.

We would now like to consider again the work of Penfield and co-workers on temporal lobe cases as, once more, these neurological findings appear to have a direct bearing on our understanding of the mental apparatus. Penfield, in his electrical stimulation of the temporal lobes of his patients, found that stimulation of certain points evoked what appeared to be memories. These evoked memories appeared to fall into two general types, the first of which the patient subjectively experienced as a sensory memory of a past event. The second type of memory was however experienced in a significantly different manner. Of this type of experience Penfield (1952) declares, 'The past seems to him (the patient) to be a present experience, because it forces itself so irresistibly upon his attention.' Kubie (1951), who has made a detailed study of the psycho-analytic significance of Penfield's findings, describes these memories in the following extracts: 'Intervals in time and place have no importance. The past is as imminent and as vivid as the present. Most important of all perhaps is the fact that what is evoked is *a specific reliving of a specific experience in life*. . . . The subject is present in the flesh as well as in the mind. This is gut memory. . . . Certainly this is the very stuff of dreams and symptoms, evoked in these instances in the operating theatre.'

This description of reactivated memories perceived as a present experience makes an interesting comparison with the reactivation of memories seen in the chronic schizophrenic patient where one is also struck by the extraordinary psychic and somatic reality of the relived memories. One of our patients showed a remarkable reactivation of her traumatic experience of an electro-convulsive therapy course which she had received five years previously. When approached one day in the group she began to shout, 'Shut up! My head has been cut off. There are enough electric lies up there to kill me without you. I am being killed by an electric shock at the back of my head. You are blowing the wind out of my brain with your electric box and your penta-shock.' While saying this the patient writhed in her chair and clutched her head as if in agony.

As we have already referred in previous sections to the correspondence between schizophrenic experiences and those occurring in states of reduced consciousness, it is interesting to consider the significance of this further apparent neurological correlate.

In this connection it is worthy of note that Kubie points to 'the suggestion of unreality feelings, depersonalization, and other dissociative phenomena' in the experiences as reported by the cortically stimulated subjects. The ego disturbance accompanying stimulation is clear in Penfield's comment that the reactivated memory is often like 'an active and familiar play, in which he himself is both the actor and the audience,' the subject feeling 'doubly conscious of the two simultaneous situations.' Kubie's further remark that 'the subject is at the same time both in an experience and outside of it, but observing it,' is practically synonymous with the type of experience we have postulated in schizophrenia due to the loss of ego boundaries. Freud, speaking of memory in 1915, said, 'Conscious memory, too, seems to depend wholly on the Preconscious and should be clearly distinguished from the memory traces in which the expressions of the Unconscious become fixed; it probably corresponds with the making of a special record. . . .' It is indeed tempting to go along with Kubie and hint that we are now on the threshold of discovering the neurological location of the memory trace. The correspondence between Penfield's reports and reports of similar experiences in schizophrenia has also led investigators such as Karagulla (1955) to postulate that both must share a focal neurological disturbance in the temporal lobes. These investigations are certainly interesting and encouraging as providing the first real evidence of the somatic correlates of Freud's model of the psychic apparatus. However, we need to know much more of the modes of interaction of psychic and physical processes and the more cautious workers such as M. Bleuler (1951) have pointed to the difficulties involved in postulating any localized functions within the complex interdependent network constituting the central nervous system.

For our purpose here we do not wish to be involved in a discussion as to whether we can locate the ego in Penfield's postulated centrencephalic system. *The point we wish to emphasize here is that in young children, where the ego has not yet fully developed, in brain damage or other physiological conditions where the ego is disturbed, and in schizophrenia where the ego does not function adequately, experiences and behavioural manifestations occur which contain elements of striking correspondence. A knowledge of these other conditions therefore aids us in attempting to cross the gap which separates us from the schizophrenic patient.*

CHAPTER TEN

Treatment of Chronic Schizophrenia

For many years now psychiatrists have recognized that prolonged institutionalization may have a deleterious effect on patients. Evidence has been advanced by Spitz (1952) and Bowlby (1951) that in young children prolonged stay in hospital or exposure to an affectionless environment may lead to permanent psychological damage. Bickford (1954), among others, has written vividly of the effect of the environment upon chronic patients. In our patients, who could be described as chronic institutionalized schizophrenics, it was impossible to disentangle the disease process from noxious environmental effects. It will be plain to the reader that many of the suggestions for treatment are, in fact, reversals of harmful environmental factors.

THE THERAPEUTIC ENVIRONMENT

The most important factor in a therapeutic environment is the people in it. Before considering any qualifications required by these people, we wish to emphasize that they *must* be constantly present in the simple physical sense. The films made by Spitz of the children whose nurses were frequently changed demonstrated the adverse clinical effect of such frequent disruptions of emotional relationships. In our experience such repeated breaks have an equally harmful effect on chronic schizophrenic patients. The first prerequisite for the nurse then is that she should be available for a prolonged period daily. Furthermore, she should not be liable for sudden transfer to other wards and activities. This requirement was met by setting up a treatment centre which allowed the twelve patients and two nurses to develop a relationship of as prolonged a nature as was administratively possible. The second prerequisite of the nurse is that she should be able to meet as many of the needs of the patients as possible. In order to do this she must be capable of understanding these needs and, the less her anxiety, the more likely she is to be able to do so and the more beneficial her work will be. H. S. Sullivan, for example, when engaging staff to work in his special ward for young schizophrenic patients at the Shepherd and Enoch Pratt Hospital, paid particular attention to the candidates' ability to understand the 'oblique communications' of schizophrenics. One may be fortunate, as we were, in finding a nurse with this intuitive capacity highly developed. If one is not so fortunate, it can be developed by training. Ideally one would prefer to follow the recommendations of Bullard (1940) and others who have recommended that selected members of the nursing staff should undergo a personal analysis. An account of a substitute method of training that we utilized follows.

TRAINING METHOD

The method of training used in this work was informal. A series of staff meetings was used to achieve the following aims: 1. To increase the nurses' sense of security and to diminish their anxieties; 2. to convey to them a framework of psychological understanding by discussions of their daily problems in managing their patients. During the early period of this work the nurses' reports were of a highly stylized form, and couched in terms that lacked descriptive content and precluded understanding. The patients were 'impulsive,' 'deteriorated,' 'quiet,' or 'hallucinating.' The first few sessions were passed in obtaining descriptions of he living individuals behind 'impulsive' and 'hallucinating.' It became clear that in fact the nurses had clear pictures of their patients, but used these terms as a kind of conventional shorthand. When they realized that their own impressions and descriptions were what was desired, they reacted enthusiastically. The following descriptions of the same patient at monthly intervals shows the changes that occurred. *First Report:* 'Mary Bruce was impulsive towards the equipment.' *Second Report:* 'Mary Bruce was standing in her corner banging a chair on the floor. She seems angry.' *Third Report:* 'I don't think Mary bangs the chair on the floor because she's angry, but because she's frightened.' Later the nurses said, 'Mary always stays in the same place. When we go near her she looks fierce and bangs her chair on the floor. She's giving us a warning to keep away. She's very frightened of us for some reason and won't allow us within a circle of six feet round her. She shouts at us, "You're sticking needles in me. Get off my name." Now that we are not worried by her shouting and noise we go up to her and speak, and this seems to soothe her.' Although at no time in these sessions were technical terms employed, it became clear to us that the nurses were able to understand the operation of mental mechanisms. For example, one day Peggy Rait struck Mrs. Alexander with a chair, and cut her head badly. The nurse described the incident as follows: 'As you know, Peggy usually helps me to bring the milk up from the store in the morning. This morning Myra asked if she could come, so I didn't take Peggy. It was just after this that Peggy hit Mrs. Alexander. I think she was annoyed with us because she didn't get to the store and took it out on Mrs. Alexander instead. In future I must be careful about patients' special jobs, because looking back I can see there have been several incidents which I didn't understand at the time which were caused by something similar.'

The achievement of the second aim, *i.e.* the framework of psychological understanding, was, of course, so interwoven with the first—*i.e.* improvement in the nurses' security—that they are really indistinguishable. As the patients ceased, in the nurses' eyes, to be incomprehensible and rather dangerous puzzles, the nurses became less and less anxious in their dealings with them.

During the staff meetings, a great deal could be done to encourage the nurses and strengthen their confidence. For example, one patient was an inveterate escaper. At first the nurses were very uneasy in case she should run away. This matter was discussed and it was decided to restrict her in no way, as on previous escapes she had always gone home. We informed the nurses that if the patient should not return we would notify the relatives and she could spend the night at home. The nurses accordingly actively encouraged the patient to leave the room by sending her out to do little tasks for them. She has at no time run away since.

Apart from such direct active support, it was necessary to ensure that the nurses felt able to speak freely at the meetings. The informality helped this, and the nurses soon realized that their observations and opinions were important factors in determining policy decisions. These policy decisions furthermore were all made at the actual meeting with agreement of all present, and no interim changes were made unilaterally before the next meeting.

These meetings were open to all members of the staff. Of the ward nurses, those from the refractory ward from which our patients were drawn attended most regularly and contributed most to the discussion. We recommend on the basis of our experience that the teaching of this type of psychological approach should always be in terms of the nurses' current work and patients. When the necessary psychology is taught out of this content, it becomes academic and the nurses are uninterested except when it enables them to pass their examinations. Freeman (1952), writing on this subject, states that there are several recommendations which can be followed in training nurses. Of these, he states, 'Perhaps the most important is an educational programme for nurses utilizing the clinical material, especially those cases which can be clearly understood in the time available for treatment.' The same author says further, 'Theoretical knowledge by itself is of little value, but constant discussion of cases compensates for this to some degree.'

THE NURSE-PATIENT RELATIONSHIP

Whereas a psychotherapist or a psychiatrist may, if he is able, see a patient for one hour daily, the other twenty-three hours of the patient's day is spent in the care of nurses. From the point of view of time alone, then, this relationship is extremely important. However, when one remembers the work the nurse does for the chronic patients, her importance becomes more obvious. She washes them, clothes them, baths them, even puts them to bed at night. She gives them their medicines, takes them for walks, and is a channel of communication with the doctors and even with their relatives. The importance of such a relationship cannot be over-emphasized and the behaviour and attitude of the nurse may often be the vital factor in the recovery or otherwise of the patient. Federn (1953), speaking of this, states: 'While every neurotic patient easily transfers from his mother to the psychoanalyst, the psychotic does not do so to a male analyst. This demonstrates how the psychotic depends on reality more than does the neurotic; that is, when he is forced to transfer his mother-relationship to a man, he confuses homo- and heterosexual feelings and becomes more perturbed.

'My contention that there should be women helpers for psychotic persons is therefore well founded, although the conclusion was reached as a result of simple experience. In all cases in which I was successful, I had such motherly aid; in some cases, the real mother was willing to help, because many women, although lacking in sublimated instinctual motherhood, have a great sense of duty toward a poor psychotic child. But the real mother is usually less helpful than a sister, or a nurse who becomes a sister.'

VALUE OF IDENTIFICATIONS

A general awareness of the importance of the nurse-patient relationship is necessary in the handling of chronic schizophrenics but, like most generalizations, it is of no practical value without a detailed theory through which its dynamics can be understood and influenced. We are of the opinion that the theory of the fundamental disturbance of schizophrenia advanced in the previous chapters gives a firm basis for therapeutic activity. It will be recalled that particular emphasis throughout has been placed on the disturbance of the ego boundaries, with resultant confusion of identity. Transient identifications (primary identification) lasted longer when the individuals with whom they were formed were constantly in the patients' environment and were making some attempt to meet their needs. In the therapeutic centre already described the nurses fulfilled both these criteria, and accordingly primary identifications with them were readily and frequently formed by the patients. One of our policies was to foster and strengthen these identifications particularly when they led to some type of constructive activity.

In order to carry out this aim it was first necessary that these transient identifications should be recognized as soon as they occurred. The necessary evidence came from the patients' behaviour, and some examples have already been given. However, in the treatment centre the early signs were rather different. The patients began to attempt to do what the nurses were doing. At first these attempts were fragmentary and disorganized, and they seldom completed the task. For example, if a nurse were mopping the floor, a patient would come and watch her, then take up the mop and make some more or less ineffectual attempt to carry out the task. When the nurses washed the dishes after a meal, the patients behaved similarly. Once the significance of these activities had been appreciated, attempts were made to encourage them. The nurse would sit beside one of the withdrawn patients and start doing something. After a time she would offer the patient similar material to work with but would not insist if the patient seemed uninterested. We found that when the nurse did this for perhaps half an hour daily for several days, the patient would usually begin to perform the same task. Often the nurses reported that the patients took up the material which the nurse herself had been using, so they decided always to work on two identical tasks, *e.g.* two articles of knitting, etc. It did appear important that the nurse should enjoy the task herself and not find it irksome and boring.

The clinical psychiatrist, with experience of the overcrowded state of the typical refractory ward, may well wonder where the nurses will come from who have time to sit for half an hour daily with a patient. We found in the treatment centre that the patients gradually took over more and more of the routine cleaning, allowing the nurses more time to devote to the patients.

It has already been mentioned in this section and in Chapter Six that identifications were more lasting and more likely to be of value when they occurred with people who were meeting the patients' needs. As the nurses became more skilful and secure, they were able to accomplish this with greater success. Emily often complained that she had no money and would ask in a perplexed way who had paid for some item of clothing which she was wearing. It was obvious that she felt she had no personal possessions and she was given a handbag by one of the nurses. This was a great success and for a time she was less perplexed and aggressive. About this time signs of attachment to the nurses began to appear. The development of this relationship could be seen in the patients' speech. Jessie began to refer to a nurse as 'Mrs. Grieg.' When asked by the nurses why she did this Jessie said, 'Because she's my mother.' It was discovered that a Mrs. Grieg had been a next-door neighbour of the family throughout Jessie's childhood and, in contrast with her own mother, had been extremely kind to her.

When primary identifications occurred, as they invariably did, it was vital to meet them with a genuine warmth and approval. This occurred spontaneously in the treatment centre, and through identification the patients gradually took over more and more of the routine work. At first the patients would only work with the nurses but gradually they took over the tasks *for* them. We say *for* the nurse because we observed that the patients did not undertake the task when the particular nurse was away, nor would they do similar work elsewhere. The patient who polished the floor of the treatment centre would not do the same work when she returned to the ward. If, however, in the morning, before going to the treatment centre, her nurse was asked to help the staff by cleaning the floor, the patient would at once help *her*, or even take the polisher from her. When for any reason the patient was upset and angry with the nurse, the activity stopped. In fact, at first the activity was clearly a primary identification, occurring only while the nurse was doing it herself. Later it developed an apparent autonomy, but nonetheless was dependent on the relationship with the nurse. It was at this stage of developing autonomy of an activity that Mrs. Rait struck Mrs. Alexander when the nurse inadvertently displaced her from her role of assistant in bringing the food from the hospital store. Sudden relapses into old patterns of behaviour, *e.g.* sitting in a corner with their knees up, outbursts of violence, and periods of demented restlessness, all occurred when another patient took over their role *with the apparent approval of the nurse*. This latter factor was the important one in inducing these unwanted reactions, for when a patient tried by herself to take over another's self-appointed task, a straightforward quarrel was usually the result without further ill effects. Federn (1953), throughout his book, stresses the importance of obtaining a positive transference. He states: 'The psychotic patient offers his positive transference to the analyst; the analyst must nourish it as something precious in order to preserve his influence.'

There were other simple measures which we found were of use in sustaining these identifications. Spare articles of the nursing uniform were left in the treatment centre so that the patients could wear them if they wished. They did in fact use these, in particular the large white aprons. The patients also made remarks about the nurses' make-up and some cosmetics were supplied. At first the patients would only use the same lipstick as the nurses; later they were pleased to have the same make and colour, but finally came to choose their own. In a similar way the care of their hair was improved by supplying them with the same home permanent wave sets as were used by the nurses.

Further changes were occurring. Patients who had gone out of the centre only in the company of the nurses now began to do so alone. The work carried out for the nurses increased in amount and became less dependent on their presence and approval. The patients moved out of the centre and undertook tasks in the hospital generally—scrubbing stairs, helping the maids in the kitchen, etc. A fuller description of the developments in this treatment centre is to be found in a separate publication (Cameron, Laing, and McGhie, 1955).

THE EMOTIONAL RELATIONSHIP

Feeding

The nature of the emotional relationships between the nurses and their patients in the treatment centre can be well illustrated by discussing food and eating. In general the nurses noticed that the patients ate more in the room than they did in the ward. Frequently the first evidence of improvement reported by the nurses was couched in terms of a change in the patients' behaviour at table. Jessie, for example, was a very disturbed person and her speech was seldom comprehensible. The nurses' first report of a change in her behaviour was when they noted that she now regularly said, 'May I have another cup of tea, please?' when she had finished her first one. It was also noted that she was stealing food from other patients, an activity which she did not show in the ward. They thought that Jessie felt she was not getting enough attention. One of them attempted to speak to her more, and this was the nurse to whom Jessie then began to refer as 'Mrs. Grieg, my mother.' The food-stealing stopped.

A good deal of attention was paid to feeding and to food because it was an indication of the emotional climate of the treatment centre. The nurses noted that when one of the patients was disturbed, she could often be soothed by sitting talking to her and giving her some milk. The order in which a particular patient gave out cups of tea was usually significant of her attitude. When patients brought chocolate or sweets to give to the others, the one who received the biggest piece was a favourite of the giver. This could occur when the patients were otherwise unable to show fondness of one another.

Later, when patients had greatly improved, alterations in feeding habits were often the first observable signs that a patient was disturbed. One patient, who had shown considerable improvement, asked if she might go home for a week-end. It was part of our policy to encourage such home visits when circumstances made this possible. Unfortunately, in this case, problems arose with the patient's relatives which delayed the necessary arrangements for one month. During this period the patient cut down her eating drastically with a subsequent rapid loss of weight. The nurses became extremely worried and anxious over this and all their attempts to encourage the patient to eat were in vain. Finally we suspected a possible connection between the fasting and the delay of the patient's home visit and explained to the patient that we were doing our best to expedite matters. The patient accepted this, saying that she had thought we had not bothered to write to her relatives. From that day her appetite improved, and a week later she was able to spend the week-end at home. In our opinion the anorexia was the result of her annoyance with us all for our apparent lack of concern. The method by which she demonstrated her feelings was certainly successful in causing both ourselves and the nurses to be acutely concerned about her welfare.

As might be expected from these observations, one of the most successful innovations was the introduction of baking. It was not only because we had noticed that the group were preoccupied with food that this was introduced but because we believed that baking was an activity in which all the patients, no matter how regressed, could take some part. The ingredients were treated as expendable at any stage, but if something edible was produced so much the better. In fact, the standard of cooking proved to be high and the quality of the patients' diet was thereby much improved. When we were particularly in favour, we were invited to join them for afternoon tea. Almost all the patients took some part in this baking; some were only helpers, beating eggs, stirring batter, or kneading dough, while others liked to prepare some special item by themselves.

General Care

As was stated at the beginning of this chapter, the treatment scheme was directed towards increasing ego function. The primary identifications were fostered in an attempt to develop autonomous functions. The need-fulfilling role of the nurses was similarly directed. There are other points in general care and administration which are worth mention.

1. *Clothing:* It was shown in Chapter Six that the habit of dressing patients in the clothing of others has a marked effect in perplexing them and reinforcing their doubts about their personal identity. This practice is well intentioned, and usually occurs because the patient has torn or damaged her own clothes and the nurses wish them to appear neat when they meet a doctor or a relative, but because of its potentially harmful effects this custom was carefully avoided in the treatment centre. We made an exception in allowing the patients to wear articles of nurses' uniform; these, and in particular aprons, were left available for them. This, as has been explained, was aimed at fostering the identification with the nurse as part of the 'ego-building' policy. It is worthy of note that as the patients progressed, they abandoned the nurses' aprons and preferred an ordinary type instead.

Some thought should be given to the selection of clothing for patients. The indiscriminate issue of clothing can on occasion be detrimental to therapeutic progress. One of our patients had a dislike of black. This was shown in her speech, as she referred to her stepmother as a 'fat black old bitch.' In our interviews with the stepmother, we discovered that she did invariably wear a black coat. When the patient was issued with a black coat from the store she was very upset and struck at the nurses when they tried to persuade her to wear it, and she remained disturbed, tearing at the coat, saying that it was not hers. On the other hand the same patient would wear only black stockings because the nurses wore these.

2. *Personal Possessions:* In the preceding section dealing with clothing we have already encroached somewhat upon the question of personal possessions. Chronic schizophrenic patients after eight to ten years in hospital have little that they can claim to be their own, and the verbalizations of our patients gave ample evidence that they were clearly aware of their destitute state. Emily, speaking as she so often did of money, would ask who had paid for things which she wore or ate. One of us used to offer cigarettes to the patients. This activity aroused mixed feelings, *e.g.* one day George Johnson, gesturing to the others who were by that time smoking, said 'They are only interested in the Hearts.' When asked what he meant by this he said, indicating the other patients again, 'They only come to see them kick the ball in Edinburgh.' One of us said, 'Who?' Johnson replied, 'The players.' There is a well-known Edinburgh football team called Hearts which had been in the sports headlines that morning and the cigarettes being handed round were Players. In this way Johnson conveyed his feeling of contempt for the others who were in his eyes only interested in receiving cigarettes. On another occasion the therapist had given him a cigarette and was trying to persuade him to talk. Johnson then told a story of how he had met a man who once bought him dinner and then expected him to be eternally grateful, so demonstrating his attitude to the giver of the cigarette. The profound resentment of the chronic schizophrenic patient against the person who gives him things appeared not merely with expendable items like cigarettes and sweets; one patient who had been talking about headscarves tore up the one she had just been given, stating that she had not paid for it.

It has already been mentioned that the practice of dressing a patient in another's clothing sometimes confused them. If the owner of the clothing became aware that her clothing was being used for someone else, she too was usually very upset. One of us who acted as observer in the refractory ward noted this on many occasions. For example, one morning the ward was unusually noisy. Although many people were shouting and upset it soon became obvious that the focal point of the disturbance was Annie Alexander. She was standing on top of the radiator shouting angrily and tearing off her clothing which she was throwing into the middle of the day-room. Every few minutes there was a battle as the nurses dressed her again; her shouted words were at first incomprehensible. Finally, throwing a shoe right across the room, she shouted, 'You can bloody well give that to P.R. too.' The initials stood for Peggy Rait, one of the treatment centre patients, who had been given a pair of Annie's shoes and her cardigan to wear that morning so that she could go down to the canteen neatly dressed. The difficulties for the nurses caused by this incident and the upsetting effect which it had on the patients concerned needs no further emphasis.

It can be seen that it is a matter of extreme importance in the general care of these patients that their personal possessions should be looked after with the greatest care, because not only are they disturbed and therapeutic progress impeded by the loss of such articles but, as we have seen, it is also difficult to have the patients accept fresh clothing without resentment.

CLEANLINESS

We have already said a good deal on the subject of the patients' personal appearance and in this section we intend only to emphasize cleanliness. One of the patients used to smear fæces on her hands, which we interpreted as a defence against the approach made to her by one of us. After a discussion with her on this subject the practice ceased. A few of the other patients had similar habits, which can be described as 'dirty.' Jim Brown also used to rub his hands with fæces. The nursing staff observed that he always did this in the toilet after he had masturbated and the patient explained that the fæces covered the semen which he felt adhered to his hands and advertised his guilt. We found that in the treatment centre behaviour of this kind became more and more unusual.

In the section dealing with the body image, an account was given of the effect on Cathy of stroking her face. It is our opinion that stimulation of the body increases awareness of the self, particularly the idea of the bodily self. There is no more appropriate occasion for this than at bath time. Our experience indicates that the personal nurse should be in charge of the entire ceremony —and ceremony it should be. Whereas the practice of one nurse attending to the undressing, another to the washing, a third to the drying and even another to the dressing may lead to speedy and efficient cleansing of a large number of patients, there is no possible therapeutic gain in such a regime, which can only increase the patients' sense of personal isolation and unwantedness.

OCCUPATIONAL THERAPY

The activities already described, in which the patients participated in the treatment centre, were therapeutic in that they were manifestations of desirable identifications which we were attempting to make permanent as part of an ego-building treatment schedule. However, the term occupational therapy is more generally used to describe various tasks which patients undertake —usually making articles out of raw material of some description. Typical tasks are knitting, sewing, rug-making, and leather work. The material necessary for this type of work was made available in the treatment centre.

In the female refractory ward one of us, who was observing the patients' behaviour there, noted that the main occupational therapy in which the patients indulged was knitting. The patients would sit and knit, usually very badly, for an indefinite time. The work often came to nothing as the patients, almost invariably, pulled the article to pieces and started over again. This kind of behaviour was noted occasionally among our patients, but tended to disappear. In attempting to find out the meaning of this aimless activity we approached various patients in the refractory ward and also some of those in the treatment centre. Their replies are best summarized in the words of Mary Bruce who said, 'I can remember very well when I did that, and why I did it. There was no one to knit for, not even myself. No one was really interested. I did it for the sake of doing something. Anyway, even if there had been any one to knit for, the quality of the wool was too poor.' The meaninglessness of the task is obvious from what she said and the practice of giving poor quality material to the refractory ward patients merely emphasized the fact. A tendency on the part of people to regard occupational therapy departments as a kind of business which must make adequate financial return is to some extent responsible for the poor quality of material which is given to refractory patients for 'wasting.' The material, however, need not be 'wasted' if it is used with therapeutic intent. The circumstances in which patients will make good use of wool, sewing material, etc. have already been indicated in the section dealing with the nurse-patient relationship. With the very regressed demented patients, the identification with the nurse was the important factor. If the nurse was interested in the task, so was the patient. Later, as the activity became more autonomous, it came to have a meaning of its own. For example, we observed that rug-making was not very successful at first. However, when the first rug was finished it was placed upon the floor of the centre. Patients then became much more interested in the rugs. When patients sewed, they were allowed to give their finished work to relatives, otherwise they were asked to sew specially for their centre. They made cushions, table covers, and napkins for their own and each other's use. The same applied to the baking, which provided an increased and, on the whole, more palatable diet for every one concerned.

In the choice of occupational therapy material we attempted again to meet the individual requirements of the patients. At first the rug canvasses supplied had standard designs upon them but later special ones were created. It was noticed that patients frequently drew a house, with a red driveway and roof, and with doors and windows closed. A rug with a similar drawing upon it was placed in the room with two others of more orthodox design. It was noted that the patients were more interested in their own picture than in the others. A mute catatonic girl, with whom the nurse had spent a good deal of time at rug-making, was very slowly beginning to make the necessary movements. When she was given a rug on which were two large red ovals with a white background, she worked much harder and finished the rug in a month. This, we believe, was mainly because red and white were her favourite colours.

At one of the staff meetings one of the occupational therapists had been listening to the account of how the patients did most of the work for them. She asked the nurses how they managed to make the patients do all these things. A nurse replied, 'We don't make the patients *do* anything. When we work ourselves they come and help us. If there is a good deal of work to do, we ask for assistance, just as one would in any ordinary group of people. We find it quite useless to try to get them to do something just for the sake of doing it. It is pointless to do that anyway, isn't it?'

PERSONAL FREEDOM

The treatment centre was run on the principle that when a patient runs away, this is not a meaningless stereotyped 'escape,' but an activity that can be understood as an avoidance of an unpleasant situation and a seeking after a better one—usually home instead of hospital. Accordingly we left the patients with full freedom to come and go as they wished, and abandoned the parole and the locked-door system. This, of course, had to be done gradually and we found that in the early days of the treatment centre, the locking and unlocking of the doors was a useful guide to the extent of the anxiety experienced by the nurses in their new roles. After a few months the doors were permanently left open.

At no time did any of our patients attempt to escape from the hospital. However, there were incidents that occurred in the treatment centre which we considered to be 'prototype' escapes. In these, the patient left the centre, usually returning to the ward. At times they did so in a disturbed and excited state. These incidents were studied in an attempt to understand their meaning, and the nurses were encouraged not to act in a prohibiting authoritative role. At the staff meetings it was reported that one patient used to go back to the ward. This occurred regularly, and at first we thought that she wished to go over alone, or to be first across. However, reports from the ward indicated that she arrived there in a very distressed condition and rushed straight into her bed. The nurses began to pay particular attention to her and watched her carefully each time. They soon noticed that she did not rush out every day but did so whenever the recreational therapist visited the centre. It appeared that the patient was in some way upset by this lady—until it was observed that in fact she was rushing out of the centre at other times as well. Finally, we realized that she was terrified of the more aggressive outbursts of Barbara Thomson who was much upset by the recreational therapist. The nurses reported that Mrs. Tyler used to watch Barbara, waiting for the inevitable outburst and, when it came, she rushed out of the room back to the ward.

Before the situation described above had been fully understood, an incident occurred which indicates the value of a liberal policy. For a few days things had not been going well in the treatment centre. The nurse whose minimal anxiety and intuitive understanding had had such a beneficial effect upon the patients had gone on holiday. The other, though good and capable, was extremely anxious when attempting to look after the centre alone. We observed that her reaction was to return to many of the restrictive practices which had been in abeyance in the centre for many months. In particular she began to keep the outer door locked. One day some twenty minutes before the patients were due to leave the treatment centre, one of us heard a noise of breaking and smashing and went up to investigate. When he opened the locked door on the landing a patient rushed past him in a very agitated state making her way back to the ward. She had been upset and had tried to leave the treatment centre, but on finding the door locked, had become wildly agitated. The nurse had not understood the reason for her distress and had tried to take her from the door by physical force and the patient had resisted violently, broken free, and had rushed into the nearby billiard room where she had broken all the cues and smashed all the electric-light bulbs over the table.

It is not our intention in discussing the subject of personal freedom to advocate a policy of total licence for patients. Nonetheless, we feel that restrictive and authoritarian practices may well mask the insecurity and anxiety of the staff and militate against any attempt to understand chronic patients and maintain them in a therapeutic environment. The feeling that the doors are locked can, in our experience, be a comfort to patients who are afraid of what they may do. A comment by a patient illustrates an often forgotten aspect of this subject. When she heard that the hospital gates were usually left open, she said, 'My goodness, that is wrong. Someone from outside might get in.' To this patient, as to many others, the hospital was a real asylum from a hostile outer world. We would conclude that it is not the open or closed door that matters, but the open or closed mind of the staff member in contact with the patient.

RELATIVES AND HOME VISITS

Although part of the policy described was to encourage the patients to go home for week-ends as soon as possible, this involved a good deal of work with the relatives of the patients, and accordingly merits separate attention. One of us throughout the scheme was carrying out an investigation of the relationship between the patients and their mothers. In the early part of the work this investigation was practically a separate activity, but eventually we came to realize its extreme value in pursuing the goals of week-ends at home and finally discharge from hospital. These interviews were found to be of value at first because of the information obtained about the early lives of the patients and the appearance and attitudes of the parents. As each mother was seen at least five times and persuaded to undergo a very full series of psychological tests, it will be appreciated that a great deal of information of significance in understanding the patients was obtained. This varied from simple facts to quite complicated stories. For example, Emily Smith used to refer to 'the fat old bitch from S—— who wore black.' In addition she used to refer to the nurses as 'ruffs' when she was annoyed with them. When the stepmother was interviewed it was discovered that she was grossly obese, that she liked to wear black clothes, and that when doing her housework she wore 'ruffs' round her rolled-up sleeves. When Jessie began to refer to one of the nurses as 'Mrs. Grieg, my mother' this reference was understood, because it was known that Mrs. Grieg had been the family's next-door neighbour when the patient was a child. The mother had said of her that she often felt that Jessie was fonder of Mrs. Grieg than of herself.

We found that the original contact with the mothers had produced a demand in them for further discussion and so we arranged a weekly meeting with those who wished to attend. Although during these meetings many subjects were discussed, we were of the opinion that their main value was the preparation we could make for the patients' visits home. The information we obtained enabled us to advise the mothers on the handling of the patients. The problems that arose as the patients began to go home were many and varied.

One mother reported that her son, whom she had been taking home regularly each week-end, was now refusing to come home with her. She expressed her anxiety over the change in her son's attitude, tending to blame it on his transfer to a new ward, although this transfer had occurred six months prior to the incident reported. When encouraged to describe in detail events leading up to the patient's refusal to accompany her, the explanation soon became obvious. During the past few weeks she had not collected the patient's leave pass at the ward but had instead walked, with her son, down the drive towards the gates. On reaching the gates she had inquired rather hesitantly if he would like to come home or have a cup of tea in the canteen instead. If the patient still requested to go home it was then necessary for them to walk back to the ward, a good ten minutes away, and arrange for a pass to be issued. Later the mother confided that her own mother was ill and that this made the patient's week-end visits rather inconvenient. She was advised to tell the patient of his grandmother's illness and, when it was again possible for the home visits to be resumed, to collect the pass at the ward and then leave for home at once. This type of problem also showed itself in the difficulties which the relatives experienced in attempting to bring patients back to hospital. They all attributed this to the unpleasant environment in which the patients lived, saying how readily they could understand the patients' unwillingness to return when they compared their homes with the wards. Again, however, a closer examination of the stories revealed situations such as this. One mother used to wait until it was time to leave for the hospital, and then she told her son to get his coat. Without further explanation she would take him by bus into the city and then bring him to the hospital. The patient used to look very sullen and upset as she brought him up the drive, and dragged away behind her. When she told this story it was suggested to her that she should be quite frank with her son that she was bringing him back to hospital, and convey to him that it was part of a regular routine which meant that he would come home every week-end. The mother reported that when she did this her son did not seem upset by returning. It emerged later that the mother felt tremendously guilty and anxious about having her son in the hospital. To her a mental hospital was a mysterious and frightful place where the 'madness' of the patients enabled the staff to treat them with thoughtlessness and even brutality. The majority of the mothers felt this, and we found the detailed reports which we were able to give them of their sons' or daughters' day-to-day life reassured them greatly. The type of difficulty described here could to some extent be overcome through the medium of such meetings.

In the later stages of the project we introduced an innovation. Patients who had improved sufficiently to travel on their own were allowed home every night. These patients attended the treatment centre from nine to five daily. This experiment has proved successful and the two patients who first began to do this have now been discharged altogether. Again, close and regular contact with the relatives was maintained.

THE RELATIONSHIP BETWEEN THE PATIENTS

Although, for descriptive purposes, we have separated the nurse-patient relationship from other relationships, it is our opinion that the patients and the staff should be viewed as a group in which we ourselves participated, although formally we were merely observers.

It will be recalled that we have already mentioned that even at the time when the patients' communications were obscure and oblique, it was possible to note preferences and dislikes for each other through observation of their behaviour. The origins of these likes and dislikes dating back, as they did in some cases, for many years were often very difficult to trace. Occasionally there was evidence that some past experience determined an attachment. A patient, Betty Cathcart, who was rapidly recovering, began to look after Cathy White, a catatonic girl, who at the time never spoke and did not move spontaneously. It became a common sight to see Betty walking along holding Cathy by the hand. Betty was the oldest of her family and was rejected by her father, who consciously suspected her paternity. Betty herself told us that she had been closest to her youngest sister whom she used to take for walks, and she also informed us that Cathy reminded her of this sister when she was very young.

The most important influences we noted were concerned with immediate relationships occurring in the treatment centre. It is at this point that the artificiality of the distinction between nurse-patient and patient-patient relationships becomes obvious, because the important factors affecting the relationships between the patients were all derived from the interplay between them and the nurses. For example, the senior nurse became concerned about Emily. She remarked that this patient was pale, thin, perplexed, unhappy, and isolated. One day when the weather was pleasant, another patient, Mrs. Faith, stated that she wished to go for a walk. The nurse asked her if she would take Emily, so both patients went out. When they returned two hours later for the midday meal, Emily was flushed and smiling, and had a good appetite. The nurse spontaneously expressed to Mrs. Faith her satisfaction with this outcome and the good relationship continued. The previous example illustrates the beginning of a relationship which was beneficial. However, the nurses also reported incidents which had an adverse effect. For example, at one stage a serious attempt was made to enliven two catatonic patients. As has already been mentioned, the technique used was that the nurses sat beside them doing something and talking to them. As far as the catatonic patients were concerned the method was a success, but other patients reacted acutely to this situation. Peggy Rait, who had greatly improved, began once again to show evidence of regression; *e.g.* once again primary identification showed itself in many small ways such as drinking tea without sugar and milk (the habit of one of the nurses). Her general appearance, tidiness, and cleanliness all deteriorated. She became more aggressive, particularly to the nurse, but also to the two patients themselves. When it was realized how much jealousy was being aroused, and the extent of the disturbance and deterioration which it was producing, steps were taken to improve the situation. For example, the afternoon after the meeting at which this problem was discussed, the nurse in question took Peggy and one or two others similarly affected into the city to shop and have afternoon tea. The following morning Peggy's appearance had improved and her speech was much less of primary process type.

EFFECT OF STAFF RELATIONSHIPS

When our work began, we were aware, in a somewhat diffuse way, of the importance of the relationships between staff members, and we have already referred to difficulties that arose in our initial relationship with the nurses directly concerned with our project. Such difficulties arose mainly in the process of communication between ourselves and the nurses. Although we were aware of the wealth of information concerning the patients that the nurses possessed, we had first to seek the removal of the barriers preventing the free interchange of such information. The stereotyped nature of the nurses' reports did not represent active resistance on their part, but appeared to be largely due to the traditional methods of nursing training which help to sustain an artificial boundary between the nurse and the doctor. In the hospital where our work was carried out, the atmosphere was such as to engender a very high degree of co-operation between staff members but, this notwithstanding, communications tended to be made only within strictly defined conventional limits. The structure of any hospital system naturally necessitates the establishment and maintenance of different hierarchical groupings among staff members, but if all the therapeutic influences in the hospital community are to be integrated in an optimum manner, there must be clear and easily accessible channels of communication between the different groups. These channels tend too often to be narrow owing to the implicit understanding that all communications will be couched in a verbal shorthand composed of standard descriptive terms that are relatively meaningless.

Through the medium of our informal weekly discussions with the nurses, such problems of communication were gradually overcome. When the nurses learned that we regarded their day-to-day observations with great interest, and welcomed their suggestions, they communicated their observations in a much more detailed and less stereotyped form. At the same time we had to guard against our own tendency occasionally to introduce terms and ideas into the discussions which the nurses would regard as meaningless jargon. Again, decisions of policy taken at these staff meetings were never unilateral but tended to be arrived at through a consensus of opinion. However, by far the most important cohesive force in our relationship with the nurses was provided by the common identifications towards the patients in the treatment centre. The nurses readily accepted any theories or ideas put forward which had a practical value in terms of their patients, whereas a series of formal lectures, based on the same ideas, but divorced from any concrete connection with the patients with which the nurse was identified, was regarded as aridly devoid of meaning. The very high level of contact which was easily maintained with the nurses in the treatment centre was never reached in our relationship with the other nurses in the hospital who were not directly concerned with our project. These observations have an important bearing on the wider issue of the training of the mental nurse, but we will return to this subject in our last section.

No activity occurring within a social structure such as a mental hospital can be considered in isolation, and this is most certainly relevant in the case of the special series of experimental situations involved in our project. The nursing staff as a whole had mixed feelings towards the work, and their feelings had quite specific effects on the patients involved. On the one hand, the nurses regarded the treatment centre as part of a mysterious and newfangled series of innovations on our part. A typical, if somewhat forthright, comment was the following series of remarks made at a staff meeting at which there was a discussion about the problems that had arisen because a patient from one of the wards had committed suicide. A male nurse said, 'There is a lack of discipline about in the hospital just now. The trouble is that they (the doctors) don't realize that these people are mad. What they want to realize is that a spot of old-fashioned discipline is needed. I think it's all because of this group racket that the trouble has arisen.' A senior sister said, 'All this newfangled carry-on will blow over, and then we'll get back to the old normal methods again.' On the other hand the treatment centre was regarded very much as a challenge. The nurses felt that they were being given an optimum situation in which to work, and the entire staff viewed the scheme as a chance to show what a high standard of nursing could do for patients. As the authors did not suggest a special name for the scheme, the nurses called it the 'Rumpus Room.' The nurses and patients who went there were the 'rumpus room nurses' and the 'rumpus room patients.'

The problems that arise when a patient is felt to be special caused a good deal of difficulty. Comments that all the 'rumpus room patients' were being specially treated were frequent among the staff. The treatment centre nurses, who did not work on a shift system but were free in the evenings and at the week-ends, were considered to have a 'cushy job.' The treatment centre nurses reacted in a defensive way to this, adopting a very protective attitude to their patients during staff discussions when they were criticized. At one staff meeting, for example, a nurse from the refractory ward was complaining of the behaviour of the group patients. One of the group nurses, after ten minutes of this, interrupted to say, 'It is only fair to mention that patients are not always encouraged when they try to help in the ward.' It emerged subsequently that the nurse who had been complaining at the meeting had been taking clothing to the laundry. Peggy Rait had gone over to help. The nurse refused curtly, saying, 'You get out of the ward enough as it is.'

Although similar situations still arise, they are not now so frequent. After some time the term 'rumpus room' fell into disuse and the nurses generally became more interested and friendly. Nurses working in the wards from which the patients in the treatment centre were drawn spontaneously visited the centre, and the nurses there found themselves being asked many friendly questions about the patients' behaviour. This change came a few weeks after one of the authors began to act as observer in the refractory ward. There he talked a good deal with the nurses during their morning break. It is unlikely, however, that this new development alone was responsible for the change. The nurses, at that time, were impressed by the very obvious improvement in the patients attending the treatment centre. Nurses are very practical people and are unimpressed by abstract theory, but a favourable alteration in the condition of their charges is the sure way to win their support. When one of our patients became well enough to be finally discharged, nurses in the wards approached the treatment centre nurses with suggestions as to ward patients who might fill the vacant place in the centre. These suggestions were reasonable and showed that the hospital nurses had a good measure of understanding of the function of the centre and of the type of patient who might benefit from attending it. Such changes in the general attitude of the nurses were of great importance, as the ultimate success of our project depended to some extent on the co-operation and goodwill of the nurses in the hospital. Many other aspects of staff relationships and the problems they evoked were demonstrated during the course of our work but are outside the context of this monograph. We have probably tended to underemphasize the role of the medical staff in determining the attitudes of the nurses. The barriers to communication between nurses and doctors are not only erected by the nursing staff, but rather are mutual constructions, and therefore can only be demolished by changes in attitudes in both groups. The subject of the effect of staff relationships in the mental hospital and of problems of communication therein has recently been examined by many workers. We were most interested to read Stanton and Schwartz's survey (1954) of 'a study of institutional participation in the treatment of psychiatric illness,' made over a five-year period. Many of the examples we have referred to are closely paralleled by the observations in this book where the problems raised are studied in some detail.

COMMUNICATION WITH CHRONIC SCHIZOPHRENIC PATIENTS

The verbal productions of schizophrenic patients are qualitatively different from those of persons not suffering from the disease. Sullivan refers to their speech as 'oblique,' and Burnham

(1955), speaking of Chestnut Lodge Sanitarium, states, 'in our hospital high informal value is placed both on receiving so-called "straight talk" from patients, and an ability to translate so-called "schizy talk." "Straight talk" is regarded as a sort of love gift, or at least a token of esteem. Often some dismay is felt by a therapist if he thinks his patient talks "straighter" to another staff member than to himself. And, on the other hand, patients' statements are often quoted, not only to illustrate the clever subtlety of the patients, but also to demonstrate the doctors' brilliance at decoding "schizy talk." '

It is our opinion that the oblique speech of the schizophrenic can only be 'decoded,' as Burnham calls it, if the therapist bears in mind the predominance of the primary process mechanisms of displacement, condensation, and symbol formation. These primary processes show as a result of ego impairment, but, as has already been emphasized, the ego always remains operating to some extent which complicates still further the communication of the schizophrenic. Lidz and Lidz (1952), writing on the subject, emphasize that the therapist's role is to translate and clarify aloud the obscure statements of the patient. This, from our point of view, is to restate in terms of the ego function (*i.e.*, the secondary process) the primary processes of the schizophrenic patient. Burnham emphasizes that in this activity the therapist must take into account the total situation. He describes as follows how he became freed from a too intense concentration on the verbal content: 'Being less bound to the verbal content also facilitated my awareness of other cues such as tone, rhythm, volume of voice, and body movements. The verbal content might be virtually ignored in commenting that his walk seemed slow and heavy and his voice subdued, and asking if this meant that he was feeling terribly sad . . . I then found myself less bound to search for a single meaning of the verbal content, and the patient's communications took on an expanded range of meaning for me.' This type of observation is particularly significant when one recalls, for example, the reactions of Emily Smith, who used to shout in an apparently stereotyped way about her stepmother. It was only by observing the nuances in tone, bodily movement, and slight changes of verbal content that one could appreciate that the significance of the reaction was markedly different from the previous occasion when it had appeared.

The role of our nurses in this aspect of the work is of some interest. Frequently, when they took some action of considerable psychological astuteness which benefited a patient, we used to ask them how they had known to do the particular thing. They always replied that they had asked the patient first. For example, one day Rachel Faith was very disturbed. She wept a good deal and broke two windows. Shortly afterwards when one of us visited the treatment centre we found her quite calm, happy, and smiling. The nurse described what had happened as follows: 'This morning there was a bus trip, and there seemed to be a great deal of jealousy among the patients as to who should go. As the average patient gets much less freedom than those in the treatment centre, it was decided that none of ours should go. As we came across, I noticed that Rachel was dragging her feet, weeping and muttering. Soon after we arrived she began to shout about people getting on to her name and about her nose being a mess and no one doing anything about it, just as she always does when she is upset. At first, nothing we could do or say seemed to console her and she eventually broke two windows. Finally, I remembered the bus trip and asked her if she would have liked to go. She said very angrily that she would, so I said that if she and any of the others wanted to go out that afternoon on an ordinary public bus, I would take them.' This remark had the desired effect of calming the patient, and that afternoon the nurse did take them out. On later occasions the patients did not react to these disappointments. They appreciated that the nurse would make some attempt to meet their wishes if she could.

In this chapter we have described our technique of treatment and rehabilitation of chronic hospitalized schizophrenic patients. Our method, while based on psycho-analytical principles, differs radically from contemporary psychological approaches to the treatment of schizophrenia. Numerous reports have appeared which demonstrate that many patients are capable of responding beneficially to a variety of techniques all derived from psychoanalysis. On the one hand, there are the dramatic methods of Rosen (1952) and Sechehaye (1951), who maintained an intimate contact with their patients over long periods, and who allowed them to relive both in action and phantasy their anxiety-laden wishes. Both Rosen and Sechehaye have had brilliant results with patients who by any standards were extremely chronic, and presented nearly every feature of schizophrenic symptomatology. On the other hand, Rosenfeld (1954), Bion (1954), and Segal (1951) maintain that it is perfectly possible to analyse certain schizophrenic patients in much the same way as a psycho-neurotic patient, although nearly all others, for example, Federn (1953), Bychowski (1952), Fromm-Reichmann (1948), have abandoned the classical technique and maintain that, even when possible, it is unnecessary and undesirable for the patient to lie on a couch and free-associate.

We believe that our method is complementary to the individual forms of therapy mentioned above and we feel that a therapeutic atmosphere fostered by a treatment centre will facilitate individual psychotherapy when it is available. The large numbers of patients in a mental hospital obviously precludes any extensive application of individual techniques, and this we feel is one advantage of our approach. A treatment centre, as envisaged in this chapter, can be combined with either individual or group psychotherapy. At the least this approach allows the chronic patient to be, to some extent, rehabilitated, in that many of the characteristic behavioural patterns associated with chronicity may be dissolved. In some chronic patients the approach is so successful as to result in sufficient improvement in the ego strength and decline in psychotic symptoms, as to allow the patient to leave the hospital and function fairly adequately at home.

A further advantage in this form of treatment is the opportunity it offers to present a practical framework in which the mental nurse may be trained in a therapeutic role. It also has the wider effect of stimulating changes in the attitude of the nursing staff throughout the hospital and promotes better understanding of the problem of the chronic patients in our mental hospital.

CHAPTER ELEVEN

Conclusions

In this monograph we have attempted to present our interpretation of the clinical phenomena encountered in chronic hospitalized schizophrenic patients. To achieve this end, we have drawn heavily upon psycho-analytic concepts described by Freud and subsequent psycho-analysts. We have essayed a comprehensive approach, following in the footsteps of Freud's 'metapsychology,' endeavouring to describe the phenomena not only against the background of the 'mental apparatus,' which emphasizes predominantly the dynamic-energic aspects of psychical activity, but also in terms of the structural concept of the ego. For us the most satisfactory psychological explanation of schizophrenic manifestations is afforded by those who suggest that it is a disease which principally affects the ego and the associated secondary process. Federn (1953) concluded that, 'The basis of sanity is correct and automatic recognition of (the) breach between subjective mental individual experiences in the world and the knowledge of the status of the world as it actually exists. Sanity means dealing with the world and with oneself with the faculty of distinguishing clearly between them. . . . It is therefore obvious that in schizophrenia it is the ego that is ill.' The 'illness' of the ego results in an impairment of the functions usually associated with it, namely the loss of adaptive capacities, perceptual disturbances, changes in the memory function, alterations in the relationship with reality, disorders of the motor apparatus, and varying degrees of loss of personal identity. In the initial stages of the disease, ego disturbances of various functions uniformly occur, irrespective of the ultimate outcome. In later stages of the disease it becomes apparent that the ego remains relatively intact in some instances while it is gravely damaged in others. In the former the damage to the ego is localized, while in the latter the ego is rendered almost totally ineffective. It is these last patients we are inclined to label 'demented.'

Bleuler (1911) regarded schizophrenic symptoms as being basically caused by a disturbance in the associative capacity combined with a splitting of the thought processes. He stated (1911) '. . . splitting is the prerequisite condition of most of the complicated phenomena of the disease. It is the splitting which gives the peculiar stamp to the entire symptomatology. However, behind the systematic splitting into definite idea-complexes, we have found a previous primary loosening of the associational structure which can lead to an irregular fragmentation of such solidly established elements as concrete ideas. The term schizophrenia refers to both kinds of splitting which often fuse in their effects.' We do not think it necessary to invoke such concepts as a disorder in the associations or splitting to give an adequate psychological explanation of schizophrenic symptoms. The psycho-analytic theory of the mind envisages a relationship between two separate types of mentation—the primary and secondary processes. The acceptance of such a view implies that the destruction of the secondary process, which can be roughly equated with the ego, permits the emergence of the primary process. It is the appearance of the primary process, now released from the inhibitory influences of the ego, which, in our view, explains so much of schizophrenic symptomatology and gives the appearance of 'splitting' described by Bleuler.

In Chapter Five we stated our basic tenet—that the condition of schizophrenia is one in which the normal continuum between the ego and the outside world is grossly disturbed. Theorists in the psycho-analytical field have long described the schizophrenic process as essentially an ego disorder. However, it remained for Federn to define the concept of the ego in such a way as to render it no longer a theoretical abstraction but a living entity, which can be subjectively experienced. He described the ego as 'the lasting or recurring psychical continuity of the body and mind of an individual in respect of space, time, and causality,' and suggested that the schizophrenic suffered from a deficiency of 'ego feeling,' or, in other words, the capacity of self-experience. From our study of chronic schizophrenic patients we have formed a similar opinion, and have concluded that this disturbance of ego feeling is the central feature characterizing the schizophrenic disease process. We have attempted to show that all other behavioural manifestations of the illness are but necessary concomitants. This attempt has involved us in a discussion of such pathological factors as the confusion of personal identity, both mental and physical, and disturbances in the secondary processes of perception, thinking, and memory. In this discussion we have also emphasized that the ego is never completely lost, even in the most demented patient, and we referred briefly to the normal ego functions that are retained and are increasingly developed in the 'ego-building' atmosphere of our treatment centre.

This last point brings us to another important element contained in our view of the nature of the ego disturbance present in schizophrenia. The phenomena described need not be looked upon as rather mysterious products of a disease process bearing no correspondence with normal experience, thus labelling the psychotic as a creature of another bizarre world, quite alien to our own. On the contrary, these experiential phenomena are experienced in many normal situations, outside psychosis, where circumstances are such as to limit the capacity for self-perception so necessary for a correct interpretation of reality. The existence of this continuum, from clear-cut ego awareness to a merging with the external environment, results in the possibility of synthesis between the observations of different workers in many fields who, using varied terminologies, have studied fluctuations in ego feeling in a variety of states. There are many difficulties to be overcome before investigators operating in different fields can extend their own ego boundaries to make such a synthesis, but we have attempted in some measure to indicate the corroborative evidence contained in these diverse findings.

We have consciously ignored any aetiological implications in discussing our views on schizophrenia, although fully aware that, accepting the conclusion that a schizophrenic state is essentially one of dissolution of the ego, we are still faced with the question as to causality. Some findings might be interpreted as implying a physiological explanation behind the diminution of ego feeling, while others point to a purely psychological causality. Our present knowledge of physical and psychical processes and the correspondence between them renders, in our opinion, any aetiological explanations purely hypothetical and possibly misleading.

The most important results of our theoretical framework lie in its applicability to a therapeutic programme that will reinstate the chronic schizophrenic patient as an active functioning human being from the deteriorated shadow who occupies a corner in a refractory ward of the mental hospital.

One of the most significant points emerging in the course of this work is the fact that treatment of chronic schizophrenic patients is, in the early stages, essentially non-verbal. This is in keeping with Eissler's (1951) comment on the success of diverse psychotherapeutic techniques. He asks, 'Is it conceivable that all these techniques have one common denominator, namely, the use of primary processes as therapeutic tools?' We do not here imply that verbal communication is to be ignored and that a consistent attempt should not be made to understand what the schizophrenic patient has to say. The attempt to understand and communicate is part of the emotional attitude necessary to allow the transient primary identifications that are constantly occurring to be retained as a basis for subsequent ego development. The schizophrenic patient certainly cannot, as Burnham points out, be understood by his verbal communications alone. To understand his behaviour and his needs, one must be aware in particular of all the interpersonal impacts to which he is subjected in the present, as well as having some knowledge of his past. The total social environment must be considered in the manner suggested by Stanton and Schwartz so that it is appreciated that some reaction by a patient may be produced by staff members apparently only in indirect contact with the patient.

The reader will have noticed that among the patients in the treatment centre there was a marked general tendency to resocialization. This was most marked among the 'demented' group of patients, and this we considered to be due to the considerable degree of disintegration of the ego. The catatonic patients required a special type of attention, and a greater degree of physical handling such as has been described, before any effect was noted. The paranoid patients were least affected, and this we believe is because of the 'successful' defensive nature of their delusional systems which reject both therapeutic and noxious factors in their environment. Quite the most surprising series of observations we made were those which first indicated restoration of the ego function in the demented type of patient. For example, the first occasion when there was evidence that it was possible that Peggy Rait might make a full recovery, as distinct from becoming a more amenable patient, occurred as follows. One of us was visiting the centre at tea-time and was offered tea. Peggy went across and began to pour out a cup. The nurse glanced round at her saying, 'Are you sure Dr. —— takes milk and sugar?' Peggy replied in a somewhat surprised and irritated tone, 'Of course I'm sure, milk and two teaspoons of sugar. Don't you remember? He has always taken both before.' This type of comment, appropriate in every way to the situation, was quite startling from a patient whose communications for nine years had been dominated by the primary processes. With the maintenance of the milieu described in Chapter Ten, these events became more frequent and finally commonplace both in this patient and in others.

On the basis of this study we have certain recommendations to put forward which we feel are pertinent, not only to the treatment of chronic schizophrenic patients, but to the task of maximizing the therapeutic function of any mental hospital community.

In essence our treatment centre simply presented the nurses with an opportunity to form durable relationships with their patients. Such relationships are formed first as primary identifications towards the nurse and it is therefore a first essential to ensure that the nurse can be constantly in the patient's environment. The standard allocation of nursing duties in the mental hospital usually necessitates a constant interchange of nursing personnel between wards, thus allowing only transitory nurse-patient relationships to be formed. In our original observations of patients in the female chronic ward it was often possible to trace the so-called 'spontaneous remissions' of patients to the development of a therapeutic relationship between a nurse and the patient. In many cases the posting of a nurse to another ward appeared to result in 'spontaneous relapses' in patients with whom the nurse had made good contact. The high nurse-patient ratio which existed in the treatment centre certainly allowed the nurses to pay more attention to particular patients, and it might well be argued that, in this way, the situation was an artificial one, divorced from the possibility of practical application to the present organization of the mental hospital. We have already described the increasing tendency on the part of the patients in the treatment centre to take over many of the routine duties that would otherwise have taken up much of the nurse's time. This would seem to constitute a partial answer to the argument that, with the existing shortage of nursing staff, the demands made upon them are so great as to preclude the possibility of their fostering relationships with their patients.

We are inclined to believe that the true answer to this problem lies in the meaning and status we give to the mental nurses' role. A broadening of the nurses' function in the mental hospital with the purpose of enhancing the therapeutic potential inherent in the nurse-patient relationship would, in our opinion, be the most effective measure to improve nursing recruitment. A new concept of mental nursing would in fact seem to be developing, and present-day psychiatric literature is replete with references to the nursing role in the mental hospital. Such workers as Stanton and Schwartz in America and Maxwell Jones in Great Britain have already stressed the need for a new attitude to mental nursing. The problem is essentially one of nursing training, which is not yet effectively designed to fit the mental nurse as a valuable member of a therapeutic team. This point is stressed in a recent report (1955) on an attempted job analysis of the mental nurse's work carried out in the Manchester area. In their conclusions the authors of this report declare : 'The one factor which has seemed to be pre-eminent (in the work of the mental nurse) is the relationship which exists between nurse and patient. . . . The whole purpose and vocation of mental nursing becomes clear in one small act of affection by the nurse, which is entirely spontaneous, and is symbolic of the mental attitude of the nurse towards her patient.' We believe that the training of the mental nurse should be such as to aid the nurse in capitalizing this therapeutic potential. This aspect of nursing training cannot be applied through formal lectures but may be developed through the medium of experience in a situation such as that provided by our treatment centre where the nurse-patient relationship is given primary emphasis. The insights and abilities developed autonomously within this framework require a minimum of intrusion by the medical staff, whose main training function is in the discussion of the nurse's observations and in the guidance of the therapeutic role.

APPENDIX A

THE SELECTION OF THE PATIENTS

The patients studied were all from the chronic refractory wards of the hospital. The first selection was made by taking all patients who had been diagnosed as suffering from schizophrenia at the time of admission. This information was available on the hospital records, and a total of 251 patients were in the hospital and considered to be suffering from schizophrenia.

A further selection was made by using a series of criteria determined before the experiment began. These criteria were as follows:

1. They should have suffered from schizophrenia for more than two years with the diagnosis established for that time.
2. They should be between 20 and 40 years of age.
3. They should have been treated by insulin or electro-shock therapy.
4. They should not have been leucotomized.
5. There should be no suggestion of mental defect.
6. The diagnosis should be approved by an independent consultant psychiatrist not directly concerned with the project.

APPENDIX B

SIX CASE HISTORIES

Case 1. Miss Myra Green (age 30 years)

The patient was the only child of her parents, who were in their forties when she was born; they have both died since she was admitted to hospital. It appears that the patient's early life was none too happy; her mother dominated the household with extreme religious views and a strict moral code. As a child the patient had no friends and later the mother's bigoted attitude made it impossible for her to have boy friends. As an infant she was difficult to feed and was inclined to be nervous, suffering from night terrors. She did well at her Primary School but became miserable and hysterical when moved to a Secondary School at the age of nine. Although nervous and shy in company, she was cheerful and talkative with people she knew well. She became a shorthand-typist and worked well until she was seventeen when she began to be very nervous and suffered from fits of trembling. She left her work and became gradually more withdrawn; finally her behaviour became markedly bizarre. She repeatedly removed her clothes and washed herself. She complained of men coming in her window, saying she was pregnant. Her body appeared unfamiliar to her. A year after she left work she was admitted to hospital and given electro-shock therapy. She improved a little and was discharged early the following year. For some time her improvement was maintained, but after the first year her condition began to deteriorate. She became very aggressive, especially to her mother, and refused to wash herself. Soon her speech consisted of a disconnected jumble of words and at times her language was obscene. Finally her behaviour towards her mother became so violent that she was readmitted to hospital in December, 1945, about eighteen months after her previous discharge. Since then she has been given insulin treatment but has steadily deteriorated. She is dirty and untidy with degraded habits such as putting her head down the W.C. She speaks to no one and sits in the ward laughing to herself. At times she openly masturbates.

Case 2. Miss Barbara Thomson (age 28 years)

She is the younger of two children, both girls. Her parents separated in 1935, when the patient was eight years old, as a result of the husband's involvement in an embezzlement charge, but the marriage had never been a success and there were constant quarrels. Since then the patient's mother has been working in an office. As a child the patient was robust and a good scholar. On leaving school at fifteen she became a shorthand typist and worked in the local Income Tax office until the onset of her present illness. She had very wide and active interests and was popular with both sexes, which among she had many friends. In September, 1947, when she was twenty-one years of age, she became very concerned over a swelling on the neck due to sunburn and complained of subjective feelings of flashings in her eyes and head. After a few weeks of observation at her local infirmary, she made a slow recovery over a period of six months and returned to work. Within a few months, however, she began to lose weight and to be rather overactive and excited. She could not concentrate at work, leaving after three months, and was admitted to hospital the following month as a voluntary patient. On admission she had some awareness that she was ill, recognizing her loss of energy and her mildly euphoric state. After electro-shock therapy and insulin treatment her condition improved and she was discharged. At home she was very irritable with her mother and became very depressed. Soon she developed the delusion that there were children running about the house and regularly went through the motions of feeding a baby. She was admitted as a certified patient at the age of twenty-five, only a year after her previous discharge. Her personal appearance has deteriorated, she is unpredictable and aggressive. She makes superficial contact and will talk fluently and incessantly on impersonal topics although displaying no affect. She does not consider herself ill and always carries a bag containing her personal belongings in readiness to go home.

Case 3. Miss Jessie Brown (age 36 years)

The patient is the elder of two siblings. Her father is dead and her mother has now stated that she wished to have nothing more to do with the patient. She was a healthy infant and easily trained. Although she was a brilliant scholar, she was inclined to be shy and sensitive with other children. At seventeen she suffered from pains in the legs and throat and was off school for a year. During this time she was irritable and wanted to be left alone. Later she went to university and took her M.A. at the age of twenty-one, proceeding to a teachers' training college. While there she took a chill and began to worry excessively about her heart. She had a tonsillectomy but could not keep up her classes and complained of general fatigue and of her brain being 'numb.' She was admitted to another hospital when twenty-three years old and, after electro-shock therapy, was discharged a few months later. She returned home but was very confused, felt that her food was being poisoned, and refused to wash. When her parents insisted on her washing, she became impulsive and aggressive. She repeatedly referred to her mother as a 'murderess' and a 'witch' and said she was hypnotizing her. Finally, she was admitted to hospital later the same year. Since admission she has steadily deteriorated and has not responded to treatment. In appearance she is haggard and untidy, her movements seem uncoordinated and she talks to herself in a rapid and incomprehensible rush of words. At times she has sudden fits of rage and stamps around the ward while at other times she sits in a corner convulsed with laughter.

Case 4. Mr. David Black (age 37 years)

The patient is the fifth of nine siblings. His father died in 1936, when the patient was eighteen years old but his mother is still alive. He was a healthy child but shy and easily bullied. His most distinctive trait was his fastidious cleanliness. When seventeen he was operated on for a tuberculous gland in the neck and became so agitated and noisy after the operation he had to be removed to an observation unit (four months) and then to a mental hospital (five months). He completely recovered and took up work as a dock labourer. At the age of twenty-two he married and has two children. His wife is a garrulous, untidy woman, unlike himself, and the marriage was not happy. The patient continued to work regularly and was popular with his colleagues. After an attack of influenza when he was twenty-nine he suddenly lost all memory of the seven years of his marriage and did not recognize his wife and children. A few weeks later he began to talk to himself and wander aimlessly around the house. He was admitted to hospital the following year in a very depressed and withdrawn state. He has been given electroshock therapy and insulin treatment without success. His mental state varies from mute depression to intense agitation. When agitated he makes aggressive advances to other patients and repeatedly states that he is dying with a bad heart. He has lost a great deal of weight, is untidy in appearance, and has many degraded habits.

Case 5. Mr. James Brown (age 30 years)

The patient is the younger of two children. As a child he was rather nervous. 'Jim had always some sort of fear about him since he was a baby.' He was a bright scholar and fond of games. Although he made friends without difficulty he preferred to be alone. He worked as a railway clerk until called up to the Army when he was eighteen years old but was discharged the following year on account of nervous illness after one year's service. At home he went back to work but had great difficulty in concentrating. He continued to work for the next few years although only as a labourer. His personality seemed to change and he began to express ideas that he was hypnotizing people at work. Whereas before he was a rather quiet, withdrawn sort of person, he now began to drink and keep rowdy company. Finally, he became aggressive at home and was admitted to hospital early in the following year at the age of thirty. He responded to electro-shock therapy and was discharged within two years at his father's request. At home he was described as being 'fairly well' for the first few months, but soon his previous symptoms began to reappear. He refused to move out of the house at any time, took no interest in things, and finally became increasingly aggressive toward his parents. He was readmitted to hospital within a few months of discharge in a very withdrawn state and has become progressively more detached and suspicious. On occasions he smears his hair with fæces and sits for hours on end silently rubbing his hands together in a cleansing motion. When he began to attend the Group he had not been known to speak during the last three years.

Case 6. Mr. Andrew Gray (age 32 years)

The patient is the eldest of three children. His mother suffered severe bilious attacks during pregnancy and the patient had similar attacks from the age of two years until he was sixteen. When his sister was born these attacks increased and he was boarded out with his aunt. He developed a slight stammer at this time. He grew up to be healthy and on leaving school worked with his father as a wool-sorter. He served in the Royal Air Force for five years and when he returned to civilian life appeared to be quieter and less sociable. Later that year definite signs of mental illness appeared and he was then admitted to a hospital for three months and given electro-shock therapy and improved. The following year he married, his wife being five months pregnant. A few years later, at the age of twenty-six, he again became very depressed and confused and threatened to attack his wife with a knife. Later he attacked his father and his mother, saying he was being poisoned. He was admitted to hospital and given electro-shock therapy and insulin treatment with improvement. Since then he has been discharged and readmitted twice with a return of his paranoid ideas. Two years ago he developed a compulsive habit of making clicking noises with his mouth and throwing his head back, and these movements, which he refers to as 'flashes,' are still very much in evidence. He is helpful, hard-working, and usually cheerful. He believes his actions are controlled by voices which make him swear, indulge in excessive masturbation, and generally behave in ways alien to his normal self.

BIBLIOGRAPHY

ABRAHAM, K. (1907) On The Significance of Sexual Trauma in Childhood for The Symptomatology of Dementia Præcox, *Clinical Papers and Essays on Psycho-Analysis*, London, Hogarth Press, 1955.

ABRAHAM, K. (1908) Psychosexual Differences Between Hysteria and Dementia Præcox, *Selected Papers on Psycho-Analysis*, London, Hogarth Press, 1927.

ABRAHAM, K. (1916) The First Pre-genital Stage of the Libido, *Selected Papers on Psycho-Analysis*, London, Hogarth Press, 1952.

ABRAHAM, K. (1924) Manic-Depressive States and the Pre-genital Levels of the Libido, *Selected Papers on Psycho-Analysis*, London, Hogarth Press, 1942.

ARIETI, S. (1948) Special Logic of Schizophrenic and Other Types of Autistic Thought, *Psychiatry, 11*, 325.

ARIETI, S. *Interpretation of Schizophrenia*, New York, Brunner, 1955.

BAK, R. C. (1954) The Schizophrenic Defence Against Aggression, *Int. J. Psycho-Anal., 35*, 129.

BERNFELD, S. (1941) The Facts of Observation in Psycho-Analysis, *J. Psychol., 12*, 289.

BICKFORD, J. A. R. (1954) The Chronic Mental Patient, *The Lancet*, 1st May, 924.

BICKFORD, J. A. R. (1955) The Forgotten Patient (series), *The Lancet*, Oct. 29th, Nov. 5th, Nov. 12th.

BION, W. R. (1954) Notes on The Theory of Schizophrenia, *Int. J. Psycho-Anal., 35*, 113.

BLEULER, E. (1911) *Dementia Præcox of The Group of Schizophrenias*, New York, International Univ. Press, 1950.

BLEULER, M. (1951) Psychiatry of Cerebral Diseases, *Brit. Med. J.*, 24th Nov., 1233.

BOWLBY, J. *Maternal Care and Mental Health*, World Health Organization Monograph, London, H.M.S.O., 1951.

BULLARD, D. (1940) The Organization of Psycho-Analytic Procedure in the Hospital, *J. Nervous and Mental Diseases, 10*, 70.

BURNHAM, D. L. (1955) Communication with Schizophrenics, *J. Am. Psychoanalytic Association, 3*, 74.

BYCHOWSKI, G. *Psychotherapy of Psychosis,* New York, Grune and Stratton, 1952.

CAMERON, J. L., LAING, R. D. & MCGHIE, A. (1955) Patient and Nurse, *The Lancet,* 31st Dec., 1384.

CAMERON, N. (1939) Schizophrenic Thinking in a Problem Solving Situation, *J. Ment. Sci., 85,* 1012.

CAMERON, N. (1944) Experimental Analysis of Schizophrenic Thinking, *Language and Thought in Schizophrenia,* ed. J. S. Kasanin, California, University Press.

EICKHOFF, L. F. W. (1955) Treatment of Childhood Schizophrenia, *J. Ment. Sci., 101,* 399.

EISSLER, K. R. (1951) Remarks on The Psycho-Analysis of Schizophrenia, *Int. J. Psycho-Anal., 32,* 139.

FAIRBAIRN, W. R. D. (1944) Endopsychic Structure Considered in Terms of Object Relationships, *Int. J. Psycho-Anal., 25,* 70.

FAIRBAIRN, W. R. D. *Psycho-Analytic Studies of The Personality,* London, Tavistock Publications, 1952.

FEDERN, P. *Ego Psychology and The Psychoses,* London, Imago Publishing Company, 1953.

FENICHEL, O. (1937) Early Stages of Ego Development, *The Collected Papers of Otto Fenichel,* Vol. II, London, Routledge and Kegan Paul, 1955.

FENICHEL, O. *The Psycho-Analytic Theory of Neurosis,* New York, Norton, 1945.

FERENCZI, S. (1914) Some Clinical Observations on Paranoia and Paraphrenia, *First Contributions to Psycho-Analysis,* London, Hogarth Press, 1952.

FREEMAN, T. Some Problems of In-Patient Psychotherapy, *Social Psychiatry,* London, Tavistock Publications, 1952.

FREUD, A. (1952) Mutual Influences in the Development of Ego and Id, *Psycho-Analytic Study of The Child, 7,* 18.

FREUD, S. (1887) *Origins of Psycho-Analysis,* London, Imago Publishing Company, 1954.

FREUD, S. (1896) Further Remarks on The Defence Neuro-Psychosis, *Collected Papers, 1,* 155, London, Hogarth Press, 1946.

FREUD, S. (1900) *The Interpretation of Dreams,* London, Allen and Unwin, 1954.

FREUD, S. (1905) Three Contributions to The Theory of Sex, *Basic Writings,* New York, Modern Library, 1938.

FREUD, S. (1911) Psycho-Analytic Notes Upon an Autobiographical Account of a Case of Paranoia (Dementia

Paranoides), *Collected Papers, 3,* 387, London, Hogarth Press, 1946.

FREUD, S. (1913) Totem and Taboo, *Basic Writings,* New York, Modern Library, 1938.

FREUD, S. (1914) On Narcissism : An Introduction, *Collected Papers, 3,* 30, London, Hogarth Press, 1946.

FREUD, S. (1915) The Unconscious, *Collected Papers, 4,* 98, London, Hogarth Press, 1946.

FREUD, S. (1919) Turning in the Ways of Psycho-Analytic Therapy, *Collected Papers, 2,* 392, London, Hogarth Press, 1946.

FREUD, S. (1921) *Group Psychology and The Analysis of the Ego,* London, Hogarth Press, 1948.

FREUD, S. *Introductory Lectures on Psycho-Analysis,* London, Allen and Unwin, 1922.

FREUD, S. (1923) *The Ego and the Id,* London, Hogarth Press, 1946.

FREUD, S. (1924) Neurosis and Psychosis, *Collected Papers, 2,* 250, London, Hogarth Press, 1946.

FREUD, S. (1924) The Loss of Reality in Neuroses and Psychoses, *Collected Papers, 2,* 277, London, Hogarth Press, 1946.

FREUD, S. (1933) *New Introductory Lectures on Psycho-Analysis,* New York, Norton, 1933.

FREUD, S. (1937) Analysis Terminable and Interminable, *Collected Papers, 5,* London, Hogarth Press, 1950, 316.

FREUD, S. (1940) *An Outline of Psycho-Analysis,* London, Hogarth Press, 1949.

FROMM-REICHMANN, F. (1948) Notes on the Development of Treatment of Schizophrenics by Psycho-Analytic Psychotherapy, *Psychiatry, 11,* 263.

GOLDSTEIN, K. *The Organism,* New York, American Book Company, 1939.

GOLDSTEIN, K. (1944) Methodological Approach to The Study of Schizophrenic Thought Disorder, *Language and Thought in Schizophrenia,* ed. J. S. Kasanin, California University Press.

HARTMANN, H. (1939) Ego Psychology and The Problem of Adaptation, *The Organization and Pathology of Thought,* ed. D. Rapaport, New York, Columbia University Press, 1951.

HARTMANN, H. Mutual Influences in The Development of

The Ego and Id, *The Psycho-Analytic Study of The Child, 7,* London, Imago Press, 1952; New York, International Universities Press.

HARTMANN, H. (1953) The Metapsychology of Schizophrenia, *Psycho-Analytic Study of the Child, 8.*

HEBB, D. O. (1955) The Mammal and His Environment, *Am. J. Psychiat., 111,* 826.

HOFFER, W. Hand, Mouth and Ego Integration, *Psycho-Analytic Study of The Child, 3* & *4,* London, Imago, 1950; New York, International Universities Press.

JACOBSON, E. (1954) On Psychotic Identifications, *Int. J. Psycho-Anal., 35,* 102.

JONES, E. (1916) The Theory of Symbolism, *Papers on Psycho-Analysis,* Baltimore, Williams and Wilkins, 1948.

JONES, M. *Social Psychiatry,* London, Tavistock Publications, 1952.

JUNG, C. (1907) *The Psychology of Dementia Præcox,* New York, Nervous and Mental Dis. Pub. Co., 1936.

JUNG, C. (1907) *Studies in Word Association,* London, Heinemann, 1919.

KANNER, L. (1949) Problems of Nosology and Psychodynamics of Early Infantile Autism, *Am. J. Orthopsychiat., 19,* 416.

KARAGULLA, I. (1955) Psychical Phenomena in Temporal Lobe Epilepsy and the Psychoses, *Brit. Med. J., 26,* 784.

KASANIN, J. S. The Disturbance of Conceptual Thinking in Schizophrenia, *Language and Thought in Schizophrenia,* ed. J. S. Kasanin, Berkeley, California University Press, 1944.

KATAN, M. (1950) Schreber's Hallucinations about the 'Little Men,' *Int. J. Psycho-Anal., 31,* 32.

KATAN, M. (1954) The Non-Psychotic Part of the Personality in Schizophrenia, *Int. J. Psycho-Anal., 35,* 119.

KLEIN, M. (1946) Notes on Some Schizoid Mechanisms, *Int. J. Psycho-Anal., 27,* 99.

KLEIN, M. *Contributions to Psycho-Analysis,* London, Hogarth Press, 1948.

KUBIE, L. (1951) Modern Concepts of The Organization of the Brain, *Psycho-Anal. Quart., 22,* 21.

LIDZ, R. & LIDZ, T. *Therapeutic Considerations Arising From The Intense Symbiotic Needs of Schizophrenic Patients,* New York, International Universities Press, 1952.

MAYER-GROSS, W., SLATER, E. & ROTH, M. *Clinical Psychiatry,* London, Cassell, 1954.

NUNBERG, H. (1921) The Course of the Libidinal Conflict in a Case of Schizophrenia, *Practice and Theory in Psycho-Analysis,* New York, Nerv. and Ment. Dis. Pub., 1948.

NUNBERG, H. (1931) The Synthetic Function of The Ego, *Practice and Theory in Psycho-Analysis,* New York, Nerv. and Ment. Dis. Pub., 1948.

PENFIELD, W. (1938) The Cerebral Cortex and Consciousness, *Arch. Neurol. and Psychiat., 11,* 412.

PENFIELD, W. (1952) Memory Mechanisms, *Arch. Neurol. & Psychiat., 67,* 128.

PENFIELD, W. & JASPER, W. *Epilepsy and The Functional Anatomy of the Human Brain,* London, Churchill, 1954.

PIAGET, J. *Judgment and Reasoning in The Child,* London, Routledge and Kegan Paul, 1928.

PIAGET, J. *The Child's Conception of The World,* London, Routledge and Kegan Paul, 1929.

PIAGET, J. *The Child's Conception of Physical Causality,* London, Routledge and Kegan Paul, 1930.

PIAGET, J. *The Language and Thought of the Child,* London, Routledge and Kegan Paul, 1932.

PIAGET, J. *The Moral Judgment of The Child,* London, Routledge and Kegan Paul, 1932.

PIAGET, J. *Play, Dreams and Imitation in Childhood,* London, Heinemann, 1951.

RANK, B. (1949) Adaptation of The Psycho-Analytic Technique For the Treatment of Young Children With Atypical Development, *Am. J. Orthopsychiat., 19,* 130.

RAPAPORT, D. *Organization and Pathology of Thought: Selected Sources,* New York, Columbia University Press, 1951.

RAPAPORT, D. (1951) The Conceptual Model of Psycho-Analysis, *Psycho-Analytic Psychiatry & Psychology,* New York, International Universities Press, 1954.

ROSEN, J. *Direct Analysis,* New York, Grune and Stratton, 1952.

ROSENFELD, H. (1950) Notes on the Psychopathology of Confusional States in Chronic Schizophrenia, *Int. J. Psycho-Anal., 31,* 132.

ROSENFELD, H. (1954) The Psycho-Analytic Approach to Acute and Chronic Schizophrenia, *Int. J. Psycho-Anal., 35,* 135.

SECHEHAYE, M. *Symbolic Realization,* New York, International Universities Press, 1951.

SEGAL, H. (1951) Some Aspects of the Analysis of a Schizophrenic, *Int. J. Psycho-Anal., 31,* 285.

SILBERER, H. (1912) On Symbol Formation, *Organization and Pathology of Thought: Selected Sources,* ed. D. Rapaport, New York, Columbia University Press, 1951.

SILBERER, M. (1909) Report on a Method of Eliciting and Observing Certain Symbolic Hallucination Phenomena, *Organization and Pathology of Thought: Selected Sources,* ed. D. Rapaport, New York, Columbia University Press, 1951.

SPIELREIN, S. (1931) in *Psycho-Analytic Theory of Neurosis,* Fenichel, O. New York, Norton, 1947.

SPITZ, R. (1952) Hospitalization: A Follow Up Report. *Psycho-Analytic Study of the Child, 7,* 18, London, Imago, 1952.

STAERCKE, A. (1920) The Reversal of the Libido Sign in Delusions of Persecution, *Int. J. Psycho-Anal., 1.*

STANTON, A. H. & SCHWARTZ, M. S. *The Mental Hospital,* London, Tavistock Publications, 1954.

STORCH, A. *The Primitive Archaic Forms of Inner Experience and Thought in Schizophrenia,* New York, Nervous and Mental Diseases Pub. Co., 1924.

SULLIVAN, H. S. (1940) *Conceptions of Modern Psychiatry,* London, Tavistock Publications, 1955.

SULLIVAN, H. S. The Language of Schizophrenia, *Language and Thought in Schizophrenia,* ed. J. S. Kasanin, Berkeley, California University Press, 1944.

TAUSK, V. (1919) On the Origin of the Influencing Machine in Schizophrenia, *Psychoanalytic Quarterly,* 1933, *2,* 263.

VAN OPHUIJSEN, J. H. W. (1920) On The Origin of The Feeling of Persecution, *Int. J. Psycho-Anal., 1.*

VIGOTSKY, L. (1934) Thought in Schizophrenia, *Arch. Neurol. Psychiat., 32,* 1063.

WERNER, H. *Comparative Psychology of Mental Development,* New York, International Universities Press, 1957.

The Work of the Mental Nurse, A Survey organized by a joint committee of the Manchester Regional Hospital Board and the University of Manchester, Manchester University Press, 1955.

L

INDEX OF PATIENTS

INDEX OF AUTHORS REFERRED TO

GENERAL INDEX

For Product Safety Concerns and Information please contact our EU
representative GPSR@taylorandfrancis.com
Taylor & Francis Verlag GmbH, Kaufingerstraße 24, 80331 München, Germany

www.ingramcontent.com/pod-product-compliance
Ingram Content Group UK Ltd.
Pitfield, Milton Keynes, MK11 3LW, UK
UKHW021956180926
475701UK00003B/54
9781138882669